The OWL DIET

Omaha Weight Loss Diet

Second Edition

CARTER O. ABBOTT, M.D.

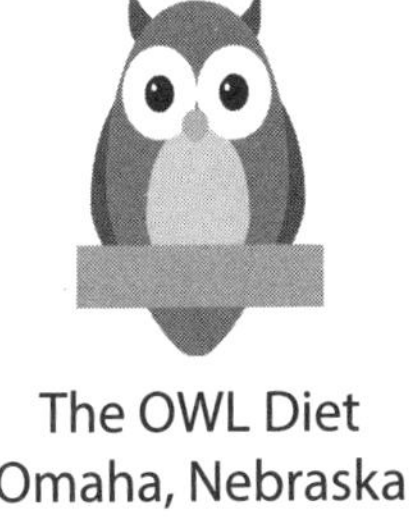

The OWL Diet
Omaha, Nebraska

An OWL Diet Publication

ISBN: 978-1-4951-5426-3

This book is not intended to serve as a substitute for a physician. Nor is it the author's intent to give medical advice contrary to that of an attending physician.

The OWL Diet, LLC
14450 Eagle Run Drive,#260
Omaha, NE 68116
(402) 614-5556

CarterAbbottMedSpa.com
OWLDiet.com

Printed in the United States of America
10 9 8 7 6 5 4 3 2 1

To my wife, Lenore,
For her patience that has no limits
For her never-ending words of encouragement
But most of all, for her unconditional love

Contents

Preface

My early medical training was severely limited in the area of nutrition. My suspicion is that, thirty years later, the situation for new medical graduates today is not much improved. However, because of my passionate interest in nutrition, weight loss, and wellness, I have taken it upon myself to become educated in these areas.

Doctors are primarily trained to diagnose and treat disease, a situation that is certainly defensible with the notion that if you are sick, you would want to be treated by a competent and knowledgeable doctor. Historically, the insurance reimbursement system in the United States has been similarly arranged—to pay doctors and hospitals to diagnose and treat diseases.

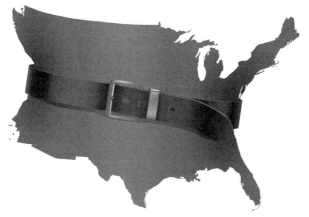

Many Americans, affected by obesity, are ready to tighten their belts and lose the weight.

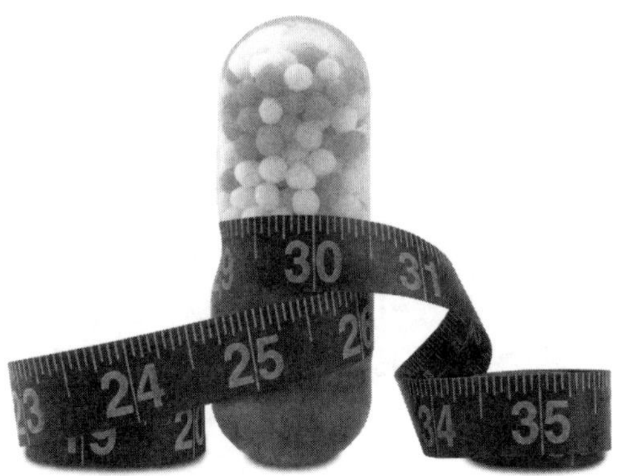

People are looking to doctors and pharmaceutical companies for a solution to weight loss.

Slowly, over time, preventative-care services have been added to the plethora of services offered by doctors and health care systems. Investing in "primary disease prevention" has proven to be financially beneficial to the patient, insurance companies, and society as a whole. Prevention can certainly have a huge impact by eliminating the personal suffering that is caused by diseases such as obesity.

In 2013, in the United States, the American Medical Association was finally successful in recognizing obesity as a disease, allowing health care providers to be reimbursed for time spent dealing with obesity in their patients. This has opened the door to invite doctors to engage in discussions with patients about weight concerns. I truly hope the conversation is just getting started.

The health hazards of obesity are well documented and indisputable. The value of treating obesity is implicit. Although it is known that many diseases are related to obesity, it is my belief that, as a whole, we doctors do a rather inadequate job of helping patients to lose weight.

Modern medicine now offers prescription drugs to treat the diseases that are caused by obesity. Blood pressure is normalized, blood sugars are stabilized, and LDL cholesterol is lowered into a healthful range—even when the patient does not lose any weight. Joints are replaced in obese patients with advanced osteoarthritis. Lower esophageal sphincters and hiatal hernias can be surgically corrected in overweight patients with acid reflux. The list goes on.

There is, however, a conspicuous absence of new medications for the treatment of obesity itself. The pharmaceutical industry has certainly tried to find treatments, but to date the results have been disappointing. The problem may be that any new treatment is only as successful as the diet plan that goes with it. Prescribing medication without offering a specific eating plan or meal plan will not work for most people. In other words, it all comes back to what we eat.

Due to the lack of effective physician-prescribed diet plans, patients have sought out weight-loss solutions on their own. Many weight-loss books have been written with the consumer in mind, and some of them are excellent. The Internet is rife with products that promise to make losing weight "easy." Dieting is *never* easy, no matter which weight-loss plan you follow.

Unfortunately, the long-term success rate of even well-accepted diet plans has proven to be discouraging. This problem stems from the difficulty of maintaining changes in human behavior as it pertains to food choices and eating patterns. I believe that diets that rely on the use of prepackaged foods, meals, bars, and shakes do not offer long-term solutions, as they fail to teach healthful food-behavior changes.

The health care community reports success with a range of bariatric surgery, surgery to modify the physical form of the gastrointestinal tract, as a way to lose weight. Whether it is a gastric bypass or banding procedure, these surgeries display some success in helping morbidly obese people lose weight. There still remain concerns about safety, long-term benefits, and cost-effectiveness of these surgical options. I suspect that we will not be able to contain the obesity problem with surgical solutions alone.

As a society, we are a long way from making the changes that are ultimately needed to curb the obesity problem in the United States. In America we see patterns emerging that potentially compound the problem. Minimum wage remains low and income disparities have widened, while the cost of food has skyrocketed. Fresh foods are often not easily found in lower socioeconomic neighborhoods. In many families, both parents work or single parents struggle to put food on the table. Some adults are working up to seven days per week to help support their family. Lack of time limits the ability to shop, cook, and prepare healthful food. The convenience of high-calorie fast foods can be appealing, given these variables.

In the first edition of *The OWL Diet,* I wrote about the reset of the social definition of obesity. Our society has developed a skewed view of what it means to be overweight. Today you may need to be fifty pounds overweight before you are labeled as having a significant weight problem. A person who is twenty to thirty pounds overweight may be considered as having a normal weight! People with a truly healthful BMI (body mass index) may be stereotyped as looking thin and unhealthy.

How do you think of yourself? Find your place on a BMI chart and get a reality check!

Obesity is now common in children and teenagers in the United States. Young people rarely feel the physical effects of their excess weight. Despite carrying the extra pounds, their joints are not yet ravaged with arthritic pain. The youthful heart and lungs of an obese child still allow them to work and play without great limitation. They feel fine, and being overweight does not single them out because many of their peers look the same.

Many pop-culture individuals who are widely admired—musicians, television celebrities, and even some professional athletes—are overweight. Clothing styles often accommodate obese individuals to allow them to dress fashionably or disguise their weight.

The goal of my diet plan is to help people attain a healthful weight and, in the process, learn a lifelong healthful way of eating. The OWL Diet is a calorie-reduced diet of approximately 800 calories per day, combined with mild to moderate physical activity and the option of using one or more prescription therapies. Anyone who participates in a calorie-reduced diet must do so with care, and I strongly encourage the regular involvement of a health care provider to supervise and monitor OWL dieters.

Some physicians object to any diet that limits energy intake to less than 1,200 calories per day. Yet, this is exactly what happens to patients who undergo the rigors of bariatric surgery: they are placed on a very restrictive low-calorie diet. The potential risks of any weight-loss intervention must be weighed against the risks of untreated obesity.

Weight-loss programs that rely heavily on increased exercise to burn calories to shed pounds work slowly and also carry the inherent risk of sustaining a personal injury secondary to higher levels of physical activity. My personal experience with heavy exercise is that my weight loss was very slow and painful. When I became injured from exercising and could no longer work out, I gained back all the weight, plus some.

I believe The OWL Diet plan is unique in that health care providers and patients work collaboratively together. This partnership of patient and physician is needed if we are ever going to be able to find a solution to the obesity problem. The plan is safe and delivers what patients want the most—faster weight loss than they were ever able to achieve on their own.

Part 1

A Smarter Way to Diet

1

My Quest for The OWL Diet

By hearing my personal story of losing weight, you will understand how The OWL Diet got started in the first place. As I reached my late thirties, my weight started to inch upward. In just a few years, I had a stubborn twenty-pound "spare tire" that simply would not go away. For more than a decade, I struggled with that unwanted weight. I really got serious about losing weight in 1998 and decided to take the advice I had given to hundreds of patients over the previous twenty-five years of my medical practice. As a medical doctor, I thought I knew the answer: *Eat less and exercise more.* Following this mantra I lost weight, but it was slow and painful. After six months of working the treadmill, stretching, lifting weights, and sweating, I was finally successful in losing fourteen pounds.

My progress then came to a roaring halt one day during weight training when I was in the middle of a bench press and suddenly experienced a severe pain in my neck and numbness down my right arm. Any movement of my neck to the right side or to look upward triggered an excruciating sharp pain from what I later discovered was a pinched nerve. I couldn't exercise...but I could still eat. You guessed it: I gained back all of the weight I had lost, and more. The neck and arm pain continued and eventually I chose to undergo neck surgery that would forever limit running or heavy lifting which might cause further neck problems.

My next setback occurred in 2004 when I tore the medial meniscus (cartilage) in my right knee while I was working in the backyard. The end result of my two injuries was that my weight shot up to 209 pounds, a 25-pound weight gain.

With obesity my health suffered. I developed hypertension (high blood pressure), I snored at night, and my knees and back ached. At 5 feet 10 inches, I was overweight, and I knew it. As unhappy as I was about my weight, I could not get past the "complaining stage" of being overweight. Heck, there were lots of people around me who looked even worse!

At 209 pounds I was still able to enjoy hiking with my wife, Lenore. During hiking trips to the mountains we were very active, walking up to eight miles a day, and no doubt burning many calories. What I noticed, however, was that with all of the healthful physical activity my wife and I experienced a constant desire to eat. We were hungry and responded to the urge by eating more granola, fruit, breads, and meats. At the end of each hiking trip we felt renewed and refreshed, but we also never lost any weight!

In 2006 I changed career directions away from traditional medicine and opened Omaha Med Spa for nonsurgical aesthetics and anti-aging treatments. I recognized that patients of the spa not only wanted to look their best, they also wanted to *feel* their best from a wellness perspective. The number-one wellness goal stated by patients was the desire to lose weight! Despite the fact that there were any number of weight-loss programs available, I realized there was a need for a medically supervised weight-loss program. If I could develop a program that worked for me, then I could offer this to my patients as well.

What I Wanted in a Weight-Loss Program

My criteria for a weight-loss program were straightforward:

- *It had to be effective.* People need to see weight-loss success. I needed to find a balance between losing weight quickly (so people felt rewarded and were willing to continue dieting) while maintaining safety.
- *It would incorporate the use of prescription medication* that could be safely prescribed by a medical provider who would be monitoring the patient during their weight loss.

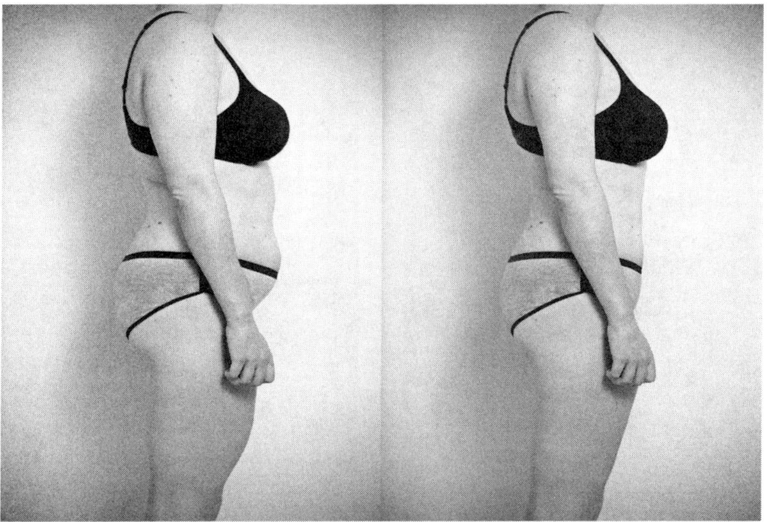

The OWL diet plan combines prescription medication with healthful amounts of food and exercise, to achieve rapid and permanent weight loss.

- *The weight-loss program had to teach people how to keep the weight off.* The more I thought about this, the more I came to realize that people needed to learn how to shop better, cook better, and eat better. Although some protein shakes and packaged food diets worked, I believed that they were yo-yo diets for most people. My diet plan had to teach people to eat better for the rest of their lives.
- *It had to allow for mild to moderate exercise* as a healthful lifestyle choice while dieting and to then continue exercising for the rest of your life. Having said that, my diet plan also had to work for people who could not exercise at all.

I started off by looking at a very old diet plan that was rediscovered and gaining popularity in 2008—"The HCG Diet." Based on theoretical concepts proposed by Dr. A.T.W. Simeons in the 1950s, The HCG Diet combined the use of a hormone called "HCG" with a very low-calorie diet of only 500 calories per day. HCG is an abbreviation for "human chorionic gonadotropin," a hormone that is produced in very large quantities by women during pregnancy. The HCG Diet had many unusual

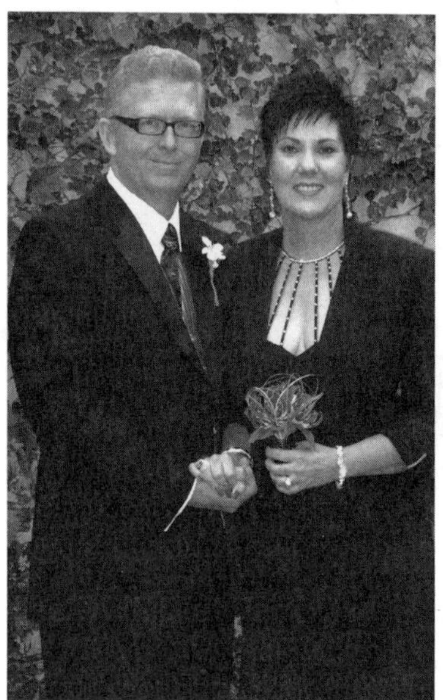

My wife, Lenore, and I before we started The OWL Diet.

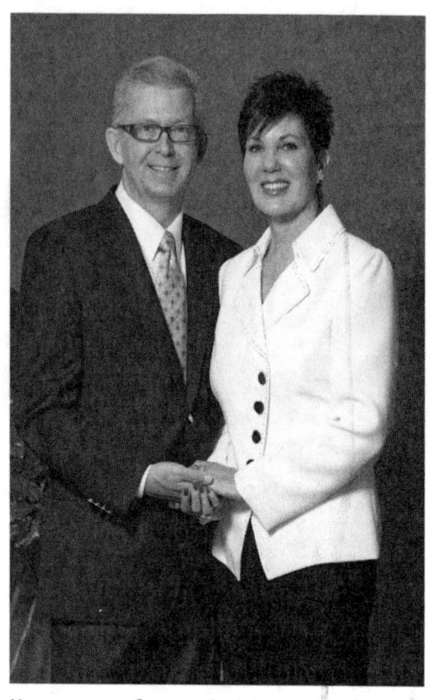

Here we are, five weeks later; each of us lost twenty pounds.

rules that made the diet plan very difficult to follow. I put aside my reservations about The HCG Diet and decided to give it a try, but only after making significant changes.

Right away I believed that the 500-calories-per-day restriction of The HCG Diet was unreasonable and unsafe. I allowed myself more food variety and more calories, and I also drank a glass of wine most days. I discarded many of The HCG Diet rules (such as limiting myself to one vegetable per day) that made the plan harder than it I thought it needed to be. On an average of about 600 to 800 calories per day, I was surprised by how well I felt. My energy level was sufficient to function normally at work and home, and my food cravings were manageable. I learned that most of my desire to eat was driven by cravings and habit, and not so much by hunger.

I finished the diet after five weeks, having reached my goal of losing 20 pounds and weighing in at 189 pounds. I felt better about myself. I even bought new clothes. But, even more importantly, I learned a lesson about eating healthful food. Eating the right foods helped me to have more energy and function better at work, and was the key to my keeping the weight off. The concept that eating healthful food would help you lose weight, keep the weight off, and improve your overall sense of wellness was so simple and yet this message seems to have been lost from our consciousness. Our bodies are designed to eat fresh fruits and vegetables, lean meats, and other food that are overall low in fat and carbohydrates.

My new diet plan taught me how to maintain a healthful weight. In fact, by continuing to make more healthful food choices after I completed my diet, I managed to lose another seven pounds!

Real Weight Loss for Real People

My personal experience with low-calorie dieting convinced me I could offer patients some real hope with a safe and effective program of medical-grade weight loss. I introduced The OWL Diet to my patients and was rewarded with helping hundreds of other people create their own personal weight-loss success stories.

My diet plan needed a name, to distinguish it from The HCG Diet, which, as I have stated, I believed was too low in calories and very restrictive. I chose the name "The OWL Diet," with OWL standing for "Omaha Weight Loss" because Omaha is the city where I developed this new way of eating. And, we've all heard about owls being wise animals! I liked the implication—The OWL Diet is a wise way to diet. After the publication of the first edition of my book, *The OWL Diet,* came out, I received phone calls and e-mails from people around the world who had great results after following my diet plan.

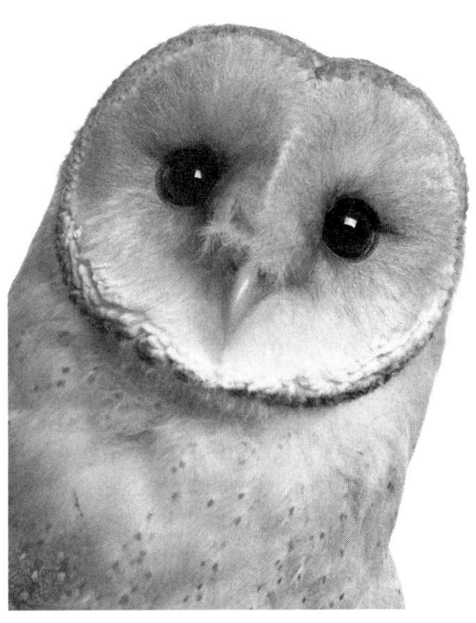

I have made further enhancements to my weight-loss program, as detailed in this second edition of *The OWL Diet.*

My changes allow all men and women, even those with physical limitations or illness, an opportunity to participate in the program.

A variety of prescription medications and hormones are now an optional part of the diet plan and can be tailored to an individual based on their medical history. Participants will also be grateful for an expanded list of food choices.

The OWL Diet today is well positioned to incorporate new treatments as they are developed and become available. My diet plan has also given severely obese people a viable alternative to bariatric surgery. I am now training other doctors and health care providers to learn The OWL Diet program so that more people can benefit.

This book gives you the tools for success in reaching your weight-loss and wellness goal. When you are ready to experience lifelong weight loss, then apply these principles and achieve your own weight-loss success story. Weight loss takes commitment and focus, skills that will also lead to positive results when applied to other challenges in life.

Your BMI and Setting Your Weight-Loss Goal

The first step to setting your weight-loss goal is to calculate your *body mass index* or *BMI* for short. The United States government has established the BMI as a standard for physicians to follow. The easiest way to find your BMI is to go to the Internet and enter "BMI Calculator" in the search bar. You will be asked to enter your height and weight to calculate your BMI. Interpret your BMI result as follows:

- If your BMI is 25–29.9 you are considered to be overweight.
- If your BMI is 30–39.9 you are considered obese.
- If your BMI is 40 or higher, you are considered to be morbidly obese.

Looking at the BMI scale, you will see that a BMI of 22–24 is considered ideal. You may feel that those numbers are too far off or too low, making your goal seem too hard to reach. I suggest that you set an initial weight-loss goal that is achievable within the first four to eight weeks. It is important to feel a sense of accomplishment for each increment of weight that is lost.

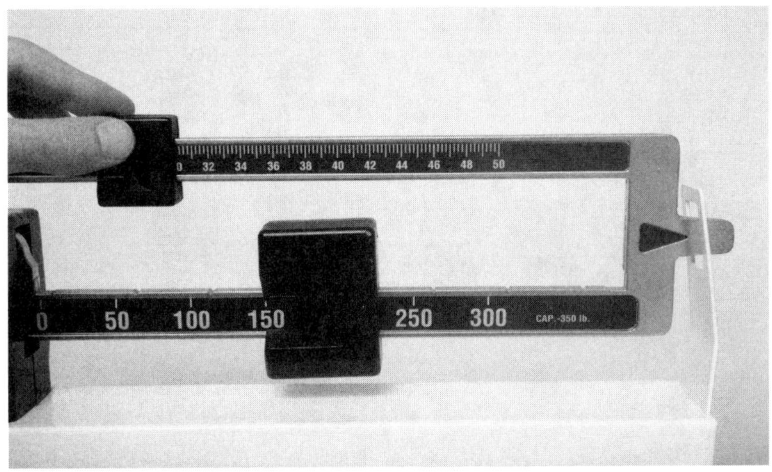

BMI is a number based on your height and weight, and provides a guideline for how much weight you should lose.

BMI calculations are only a guide. The BMI scale does not take into account different body build, muscle mass, age, or gender. I have found that if you are under 5'3" or over 6'0", modifications are often needed and a BMI of 25 to 26 may be a more realistic goal.

Some people prefer to set a goal based on percentage of body fat. Others are more interested in subjective goals such as "How I look in my clothes."

Work with a health care provider to set your goal weight. Medical-grade dieting, which incorporates the use of medically supervised prescription medication, should be limited to participants who are overweight and typically have a BMI of 25 or higher.

How Fast Will I Lose Weight?

Typically, you will lose the most weight during your first week on The OWL Diet. A common mistake is to then set the bar too high for subsequent weeks. For example, "I lost six pounds the first week, so that should be my goal every week." That is an unrealistic goal and it will certainly set you up for failure. Every week on The OWL Diet you need to look at your overall weight-loss progress since you started the program.

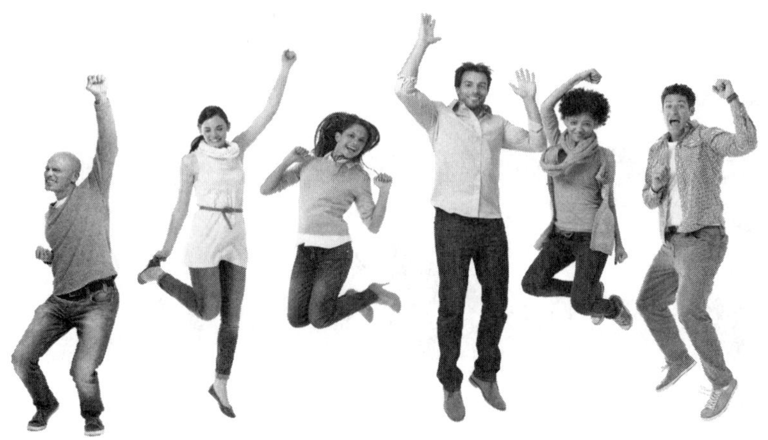

The OWL Diet works, and you will feel great once you reach your goal weight.

Be aware that men, young people, tall people, and people who have the most weight to lose often lose weight faster. The average weight loss observed per month is 15 pounds for women and 20 pounds for men. These numbers are an approximation and vary between individuals. If you are a seventy-year-old female with a height of 5'0" then losing at a rate of 8–10 pounds a month would be an excellent result. A young person who starts at more than 275 pounds will often lose 25–30 pounds the first month, but they won't keep losing at that rate. As you get closer to your weight-loss goal, your rate of weight loss will slow.

The OWL Diet participants who have lost 100 pounds typically took six months or longer to achieve that goal. If you are a sixty-five-year-old woman who wants to lose 20 pounds, it is not going to happen in one month. A more realistic goal is to lose 20 pounds over two months.

Losing weight is not a race! It is a journey, and the final goal is to keep the weight off permanently. Do not be in too much of a hurry to lose weight. It will take some time. What would be the point of losing 30 pounds in 30 days only to gain it all back again when you cannot maintain the pace? Take it a week at a time, and you will be pleasantly surprised with your success.

You Are Not Perfect

The perfect OWL Diet participant would follow the program flawlessly, eating exactly the right amounts that are allowed each and every day and not breaking any rules. So far I have not met anyone who has followed the diet plan perfectly every single day. We all have flaws and imperfections. To succeed on any diet, you will need to overcome perfectionism.

Following are some helpful things to say to yourself to overcome perfectionism:

- No one is totally perfect, and neither am I.
- I will strive to do my best, and be content with my success every week on the diet.
- Making a mistake on the diet does not mean I am a failure, and does not mean that I have to quit.
- I will do my best, because I really want to achieve my weight-loss goal, but I will avoid placing undue pressure on myself to be perfect.
- I will set realistic goals that I can accomplish.
- Friends and family who are important to me will accept my imperfections, as long as they know I have trying my hardest.

Self-Esteem

Self-esteem and self-worth are a measure of how much we like and value who we are. Self-esteem develops over time and is influenced by our personal history, thoughts, and feelings.

Many people who are overweight have lower self-esteem than they would like. One of the best ways to build self-esteem is to succeed, and The OWL Diet is a great beginning!

Motivation Self-Assessment

At this point I would like you to pause and reflect on what I have shared with you so far. Take time to read the following questions, and be honest with yourself as you answer them. You may even want to write down your answers so you can go back and read them later. This is your starting point, and along your journey to weight loss it may prove helpful to go back and review these questions and your answers as a way to stay on track with The OWL Diet.

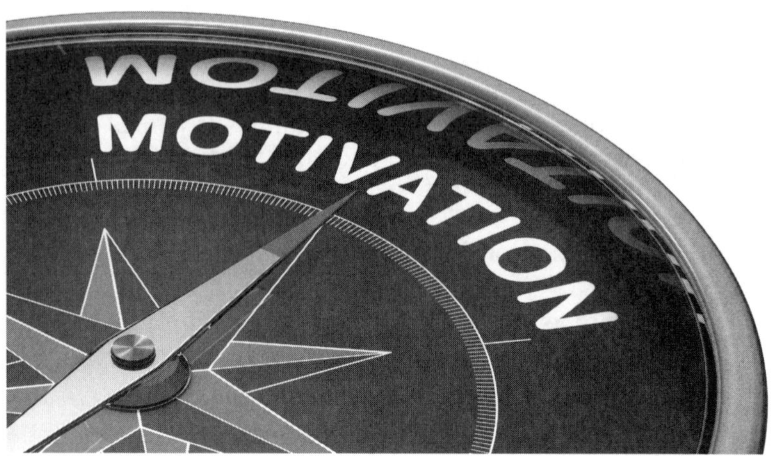

Motivation is the engine that keeps you moving in the right direction during your weight loss journey.

- What is your motivation to lose weight?
- Are you past the "complaining stage"?
- Are you ready to regain control over your weight, and keep your weight off forever?
- What is your weight-loss goal?
- How long do you think it will take you to reach that goal?
- Are you prepared to take a break from dieting if needed?
- Who will be supportive of your effort to lose weight?
- Who may not be supportive, and might even try to sabotage your success at dieting? And how should you react to them?

2

How Is The Owl Diet Different?

Most of the people who have come to me for help in losing weight report that they have already tried many diet plans. Even when a diet worked (they lost weight) they found that they gained all of the weight back again.

To be effective, The OWL Diet needed to offer a new approach to losing weight and keeping it off. The OWL Diet strikes the right balance between losing weight quickly and maintaining safety. This chapter explains the features of my plan: eating realistic portions of healthful food, putting yourself under medical supervision while you diet, allowing the use of prescription medications, and maintaining mild to moderate exercise.

Weight Loss that Is Fast, Safe, and Life-Changing

There are some diet programs that promote healthful eating habits, but often the rate of progress is slow, with participants losing one to two pounds per week. Although this is fine if you need to lose only about ten pounds, I found that the average weight-loss goal is much higher—typically around fifty pounds. People feel that they need to lose weight at a faster rate for them to stay motivated to continue with the diet plan.

I have observed that it is harder for women to lose weight compared to men. Women usually have a lower metabolic rate and their weight is often negatively impacted by pregnancy and hormonal changes that occur over the course of their lifetime. The group of people who appear to need the greatest amount of help are women after the age of thirty-five. They often report that they had tried unsuccessfully on their own to lose weight, using a combination of reducing calories and increasing exercise. They often complain of very slow to no weight loss, even though they are following healthful guidelines provided by wellness experts.

As mentioned earlier, the average weight loss on The OWL Diet is approximately 15 pounds per month for women and 20 pounds per month for men. At this rate of weight loss, patients, including those who need to lose more than 100 pounds, generally remain motivated to keep working toward their weight goals. This fact allows The OWL Diet results to compare favorably to the surgical option for losing weight, generally known as bariatric surgery.

I went on the OWL Diet and I couldn't believe how easy it was to lose twenty pounds in just five weeks. I am very satisfied with this diet plan.
Jane, 64

Patients who lose weight on The OWL Diet do not have to face the inherent risks associated with bariatric surgery, hospital stays, and postoperative complications. Although medically supervised OWL Diet participation also comes at financial expense to the patient, the cost of losing weight following my nonsurgical diet plan is considerably more affordable than bariatric surgery. I tell patients that if they follow the plan, lose weight, and make it a lifelong goal to eat better, then this is likely the best investment they will ever make.

I have seen patients who have lost weight through bariatric surgery, only to start gaining it back again. They see me several years after their surgery with the need to get back to the basics about eating healthful foods in appropriate portions. That is what lifelong weight control is all about—eating better.

The OWL Diet delivers the results that patients are looking for: losing weight quickly and safely. By learning to shop, cook, and eat better, they are on the path toward achieving a healthful, lifelong weight.

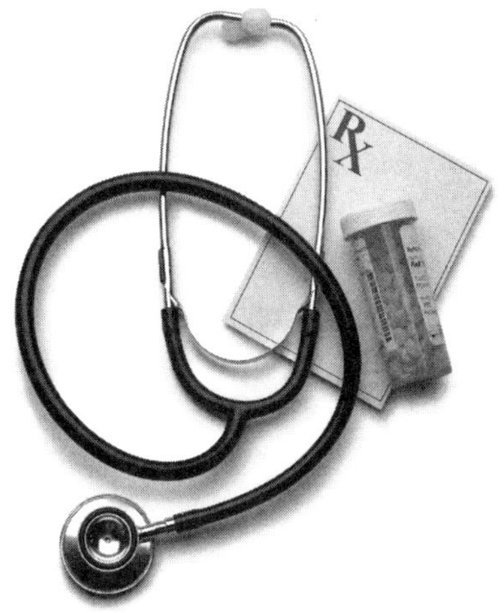

The OWL Diet is a medical-grade weight loss program.

Partnership with Health Care Providers

With a reduced-calorie intake of approximately 800 calories per day on The OWL Diet, participants are directed to be seen regularly by a health care provider. As mentioned earlier, success on The OWL Diet is enhanced by utilizing appropriate prescription medications and hormones that are only available from medical doctors and, in some states, also from mid-level practitioners (known as nurse practitioners and physician assistants).

The health care provider helps ensure your safety and success by monitoring your:

- Weight and blood pressure (and blood sugars as needed)
- Compliance with eating the correct types and amounts of food daily, spaced out over the course of the day
- Compliance with maintaining adequate hydration with water
- Practicing mild to moderate physical activity
- Avoiding excessive physical activity that is not recommended on a reduced-calorie diet
- Using prescription medications correctly
- Having any potential side effects from treatment

- Regular bowel movements
- Getting an adequate amount of sleep

This partnership with a health care provider is an important part of OWL Diet success. Health care providers and patients work cooperatively together to improve your overall health and wellness.

Who Can Succeed with The OWL Diet

Men and women with a range of medical histories may all achieve success with OWL dieting. The OWL Diet is customizable for each patient, based on their health history. This allows all people to participate in my diet plan. For example, patients with different cancer histories can all participate, but they may be more limited in range of prescribed therapies that will be made available to them.

Although I encourage mild to moderate physical activity, I have also had success helping people lose weight whose ability to exercise is very limited due to their current health problems. Examples have included patients with joint arthritis or neurological diseases such as multiple sclerosis.

I have had patients who have achieved excellent success on The OWL Diet plan without the use of any prescribed therapies. Prescribed therapies are optional and subject to informed choices made by the patient after consultation with their health care provider. Not all patients will qualify for the use of all of the different prescribed therapies.

3

The Keys to Success

There are no magic bullets in dieting. The key to success on The OWL Diet is to follow the diet plan exactly. Dieting is never easy, but if you learn The OWL Diet and follow it faithfully then it will work for you. The OWL Diet does not fail people, but people will fail The OWL Diet. Success depends on focus, determination, commitment, and patience.

As you read this chapter detailing some of the keys to successful OWL dieting, think about how they apply to you personally.

Understanding Hunger, Food, and Your Behavior

Most of us no longer eat to survive. We eat out of habit. We eat of out boredom. We eat for comfort. We eat because we are worried or stressed or unhappy. We eat because we are addicted to sugar and salt. We eat because there is a tempting array of foods readily available that are fast and affordable. On that list are junk foods and highly processed foods laden with salt, sugars, and preservatives. We still call them "food" but they are anything but fresh and nutritious.

Our ancestors would be amazed by the variety of foods that are now available in the average American supermarket. For most of human history we needed to hunt and gather wild foods to survive. It was a full-time job for both man and woman to stalk game and gather and cook edible plants, roots, seeds, nuts, and berries. Only those who were able to provide for themselves and their families survived, ensuring a strengthening human race of resourceful and capable hunters and gatherers. Hunters and gatherers certainly were not prone to obesity!

Unlike the eras when our ancestors spent days tracking animals, searching for edible plants, or toiling in their fields, we modern humans can get an absurd abundance of food simply by strolling down the aisles of our local supermarkets. We no longer have to exert the same energy to acquire food.

I have tried every diet you can imagine, and I have never been able to keep the weight. But, I have lost 47 pounds in ten weeks on The OWL Diet and have kept the weight off. Also, this program has taught me how to eat properly.
Heidi, 38

Worse yet, fast food provides affordable, high-calorie food choices that have become a staple of our diet, much to our detriment. Fast food is often the major source of nutrition in poor communities where supermarkets and more healthful food choices are an expensive bus or cab ride away.

In rural areas, the labor involved in growing food has been greatly reduced by mechanization. Whereas farmers of fifty years ago were rarely overweight, it is now commonplace to see obesity reaching into rural communities. Mechanization has progressed, but in many ways eating habits have not changed to adjust to a lower output of personal energy needed to harvest the food from the farm.

You can see where all of this is leading—we work less to obtain more food. And the result is we have become an obese society.

Our social structure today also promotes overeating. With many families relying on two incomes, the trend is to "dine out" due to time constraints. Children raised thirty years ago were fortunate to receive a weekly allowance that permitted a rare trip to the local store for a small amount of candy. Children today often have access to disposable incomes that allow them daily access to fast food, candy, and soft drinks outside the family home and school. Prepared foods such as fried chicken and pizza were once a major treat for a family, but have now

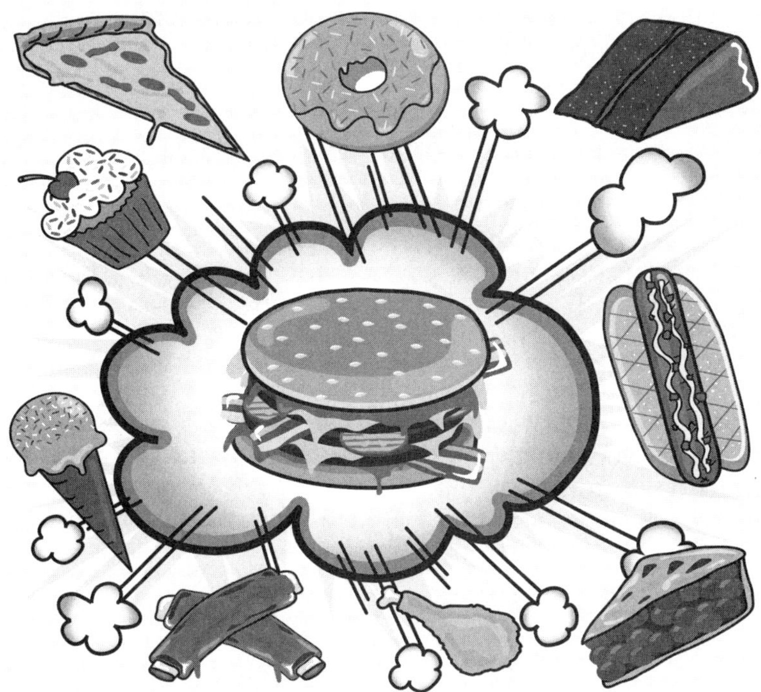

Our diet is too high in sugar, carbs, and cooking oil—we need to break the habit.

become a regular part of our eating habit and, sadly, they are often a part of the daily school lunch menu.

We have also become habitual consumers of junk food. I hesitate to call it "food," because these highly processed concoctions no longer resemble the kind of food that just a century ago was harvested and eaten fresh. We eat these products because we like them. Actually, we love them. We are addicted to them and we eat them not for survival but for pleasure.

We all have a survival instinct to feel hunger and search for a source of food, because the consumption of food is a vital component of our continued existence. Food is the energy that fuels the body. When we are genuinely hungry, the act of eating then triggers the release of chemical transmitters in the brain that make us feel more content. But we don't have to be hungry to obtain that positive feedback that food provides us with.

It is then easy to see why eating during times of emotional stress may initially relieve some of the emotional discomfort. Stress can lead us to eat compulsively and repetitively even when our stomach tells us we are full. At some point during the eating binge the positive feedback from food stops, and we then experience feelings of despair, hopelessness, and self-hatred.

The recipe for an obese society is the lethal combination of sedentary jobs, increased time with technology (phones, computers and TVs), and the avalanche of readily available junk food.

Motivation

What is your motivation to lose weight? A quick answer of "I am overweight, isn't that enough of a reason?" probably won't do. You need to dig inside yourself a bit deeper to find sources of motivation that will help drive you to obtain your goal weight.

Avoiding Health Problems

Perhaps you have been told by your health care provider that you need to lose weight. The warning may have come before a health problem develops. Perhaps you feel fine, are on no medications, but know that your weight places you at a high risk of developing a health problem such as diabetes or heart disease. Losing weight to keep your doctor happy is not enough of a motivator. Maybe wanting to be around to see your children get married and to spend time with grandchildren is a greater motivator. Or perhaps you have seen relatives suffer from the complications of heart disease or diabetes and want to avoid similar problems.

If you have not heeded conventional wisdom to "lose weight now to prevent health problems later," then you may find yourself already suffering from one of the many diseases that are driven by obesity, such as diabetes and heart disease. As a diabetic, you may have complications with your eyes, kidneys, leg circulation, or sexual function. With a heart problem, you may find it hard to climb stairs, your breathing is short-winded, or your legs are swelling.

Improving Appearance

Another motivating factor may be your appearance standing naked in front a mirror, in photographs, or in bed with your partner. The way we feel about our outward appearance can have a strong impact on self-confidence and self-worth. Lacking in self-esteem often negatively impacts our personal relationships and our success at work.

Planning for Upcoming Events

Upcoming special events often motivate people to shed a few pounds. It may be a high school reunion, family reunion, beach vacation, or big birthday. Family weddings and the knowledge that photos will be taken and shared with many people can also influence the decision to diet. My experience has been that any one of these events can have a major positive effect on diet success, but the success frequently gives way to regaining the weight a short time later. If you lose weight for a special event, make a point of working to keep the weight off permanently.

I am so impressed with my results of The OWL Diet. It's been worth every penny! Dr. Abbott's staff are so caring and attentive to my needs. They are always available for my questions and concerns.

Mary, 47

"Reinventing" Yourself

Unscheduled changes in their lives can also propel people to decide to lose weight. Common examples are the end of a long-term relationship (marriage or partner) caused by divorce or illness. These life changes often cause us to reinvent who we are, and that includes how we physically appear when seen by others. The desire to find a new companion is a strong motivator to make personal improvements that include achieving a more healthful weight.

Being overweight or obese may make you feel that others judge you before they get to know you. You may feel labeled or categorized in ways that do not reflect the person that you know yourself to be. These stereotypes, although unfair, are commonplace and create barriers to meeting other people and may impact your career opportunities as well as your social life.

Losing weight for other people in your life is not usually successful. You cannot lose weight for your friend, partner, spouse, or parent—you must lose it for yourself.

Motivation Leads to Change

Motivation inspires an individual to change their behavior and take action toward achieving a desired goal. To achieve that goal (in this case, losing weight) you must understand the steps you need to take to make that "change" (succeeding on The OWL Diet plan).

Considering Change

There are stages in losing weight. The first step is to *consider change.* I call this "getting past the complaining stage." Most of us complain about our weight for quite some time before we get to the point that we become motivated enough to make a change and find a diet plan that will work for us. Waiting for motivation to be strong enough to make us initiate change may sometimes be a long wait.

Deciding to Change

The next step is to *make the decision to change.* You have already reached this point because you are reading the book, and, in order to follow The OWL Diet, will be seeing a health care provider who will help guide you through the process. You are weighing your options, but you have decided you want to make a change.

Making the Change

Then you actually *make change happen.* You will learn the diet, follow it the best that you can, and achieve your weight-loss goal. Ongoing motivation to succeed will be vital over the weeks that follow on your weight-loss journey. If you lose motivation, you will lose focus and your success will be less than you wanted.

Maintaining the Change

The final step is to *maintain the change*. Now that you have lost the weight, you need to draw on the desire and motivation to keep it off forever. Most people call this the "maintenance" part of the weight-loss plan.

The above steps are familiar to people who have overcome addiction. The same mental skill set is needed to master control over our weight and live a healthier life by losing the weight and keeping it off permanently. What step are you at right now?

During your weight-loss journey you need to do sustain your motivation to succeed. Trust me, there will be times over the coming weeks and months that your motivation will be challenged. Without a strong motivation to continue, you will lose focus and you may stop dieting.

Timing: Finding the Right Time for Weight Loss

Once you feel motivated to lose the weight, and understand the changes that you will need to make, you then need to select the correct time to start the diet plan. Timing for success is critical, especially for the first month of dieting. You want to set yourself up for success the first month, which will in turn propel you toward your ultimate goal.

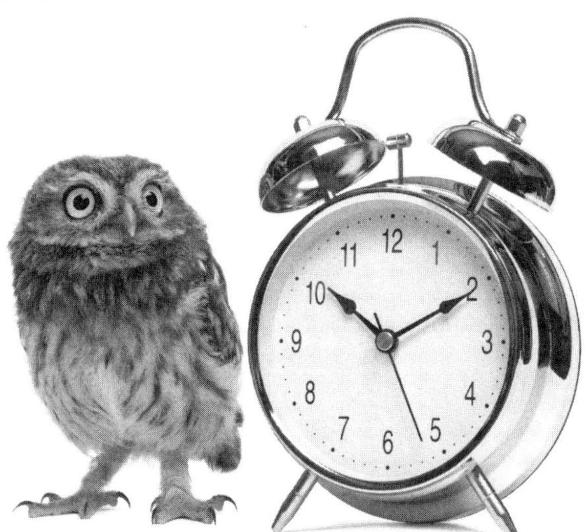

Timing is important. Start The OWL Diet at a time that will ensure your success.

Look at the calendar from a personal perspective. Are there birthdays, anniversaries, graduations, holidays, or vacations coming up in the next month? If so, you may need to start your diet plan after the event.

Do you have travel demands for your work? Do you need to spend nights away from home as part of your job? Do you need to eat meals as a part of conducting business?

There may be some of you who say, "I am always busy and there is never a good time to start a new diet." This may be true, but don't let this excuse cause you to put off dieting until it is too late. You must choose the *best possible* time for starting.

Prescription Medication

One of the key benefits of The OWL Diet plan is the option to use one or more prescribed therapies. They may be a combination of medications and hormones. Some people may need only one of the prescription options; others need to utilize up to all five of the treatments described in this book. Prescription treatments that are currently available include:

- phentermine
- topiramate
- testosterone
- human chorionic gonadotropin (HCG)
- vitamin B-12 injections

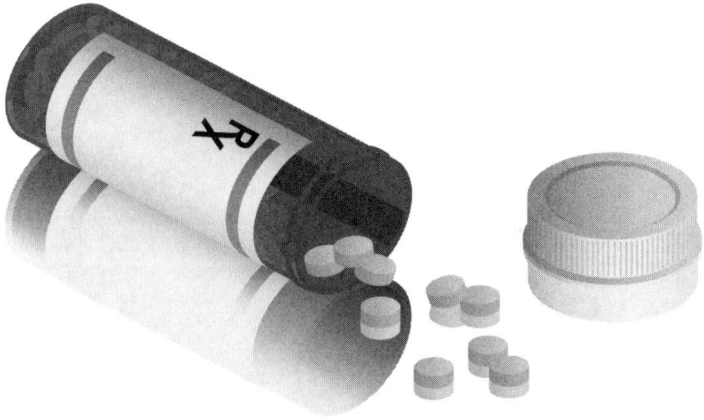

Your doctor may prescribe prescription drugs, appetite suppressants, to help you lose weight.

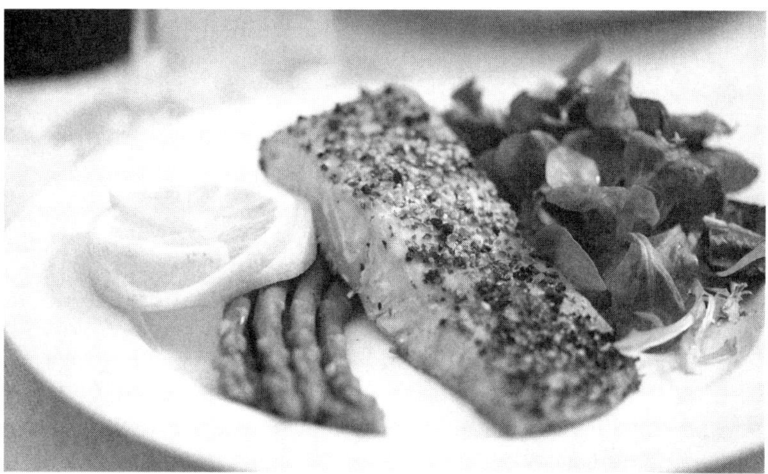

The OWL Diet teaches to eat smaller portions—up to 7 ounces of lean meat, four cups of fresh vegetables, and three servings of fruit. You may exchange one fruit for an 80-calorie serving of yogurt.

You will learn the specifics of each of the five therapies in chapter 4. Some treatments may not be suitable for your use, based on your medical history. For example, a patient who has a history of substance abuse, heart palpitations, or anxiety attacks is not a candidate for use of phentermine. Topiramate should be used with caution in women who are still in their reproductive years due to the risk of fetal injury. HCG use is often avoided in women who have had a history of breast cancer.

Relying on the prescription medication alone will not result in weight-loss success. The OWL Diet is most successful with the proper use of prescription medications combined with eating foods that are allowed on the program.

Your journey to weight loss will be more difficult without the help of prescription medications. But if you follow the low-calorie diet as described in this book, even without the benefit of using any prescription treatments you will still lose weight. This is a simple reality of arithmetic and metabolism. Your body is like a furnace that consumes energy. The energy is measured in calories and the body needs to burn a certain amount of calories per day to maintain life. If the intake of food calories is less than what the "furnace" needs to burn every day, the body will burn fat as a source of more calories.

If you undertake The OWL Diet without the use of prescription treatments, I still strongly advise you to see a health care worker every week. The visit helps you stay accountable to yourself, and it also gives the health professional an opportunity to check your weight and blood pressure and inquire about any other medical issues you may be dealing with.

OWL Rules for Success

It has been my experience that people who try to diet without coaching, support, and medical monitoring tend to have limited success. The greatest risk occurs from people who feel they are following the program, but in fact may not be eating the right foods and staying hydrated. The OWL Diet has several specific rules that must be adhered to, and they are primarily the following:

- Eating a large variety of foods from different food groups
- Spreading the food across three meals and three snacks per day
- Engaging in mild to moderate exercise but not more than that

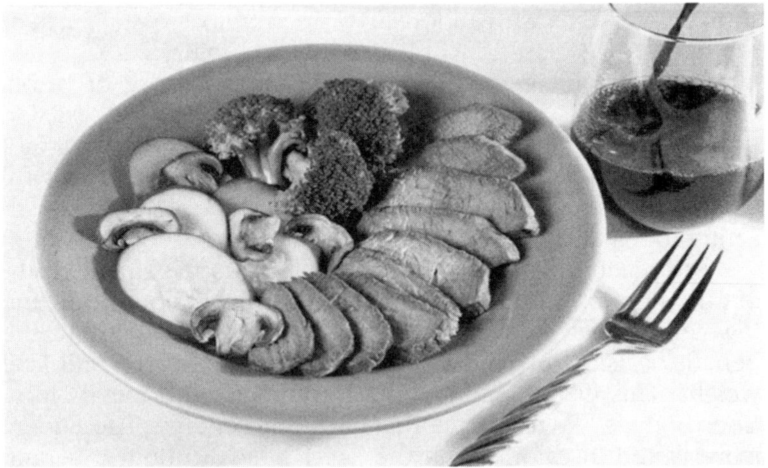

Strive to eat a variety of foods while you're on The OWL Diet. Variety and flavors (seasonings) will make mealtime more enjoyable.

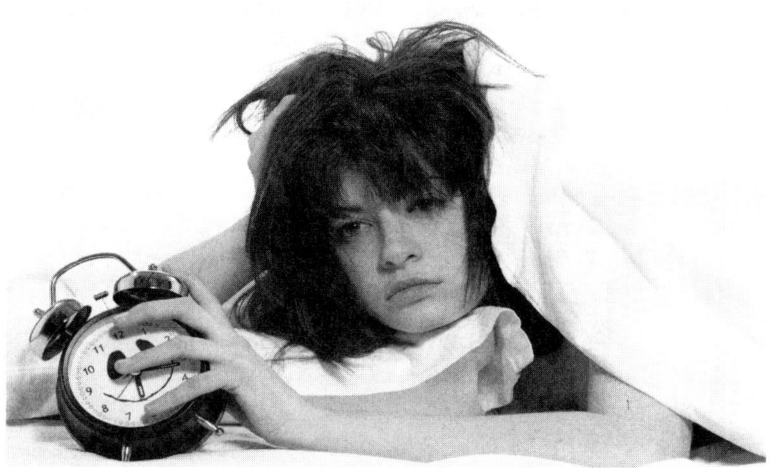

Getting an adequate amount of sleep will help you manage your hunger and food cravings.

- Staying well hydrated over the course of the day
- Obtaining an adequate amount of sleep
- Maintaining regular bowel patterns
- Taking the correct amounts of vitamins and supplements

Meal Planning

In Part Three of this book, The Complete OWL Diet Plan, I provide detailed information about the food options available on The OWL Diet. I believe you will be pleasantly surprised to find a long list of foods to choose from. By offering a wide variety of food choices, you will never get bored on The OWL Diet plan. Perhaps even more importantly, this way of eating will teach you how to continue to make healthful food choices as part of maintenance eating after you have reached your goal weight.

Your job will be to select the specific food items that you like best from the long list of approved food items I provide. Meal planning means how you arrange the foods over the course of a day. You must select allowed food only, and combine them in the correct portions to create three meals and three snacks every day.

Spreading your food out over the course of each day will control your hunger, stimulate your metabolism, and help ensure wellness during your weight-loss journey. In maintenance, you must continue to abide by this healthful practice of eating and drinking during the course of every day.

Following are some examples of meal planning that would work on The OWL Diet. I provide you with specific brand names to help you find these products in the grocery store. As an example, Walden Farms provides a wide variety of calorie-free food options that include salad dressings and BBQ sauce.

Example 1: Daily Meal Plan

Breakfast:

½ cup total of raw vegetables (mushroom, red peppers, and onions) pan-fried using PAM spray and combined with ¼ cup of Egg Beaters, then pan-fried to make an omelet. Season to taste and place on a toasted ½ Bagel Thin. Beverages: coffee and a tall glass of water containing fresh lemon juice and Splenda.

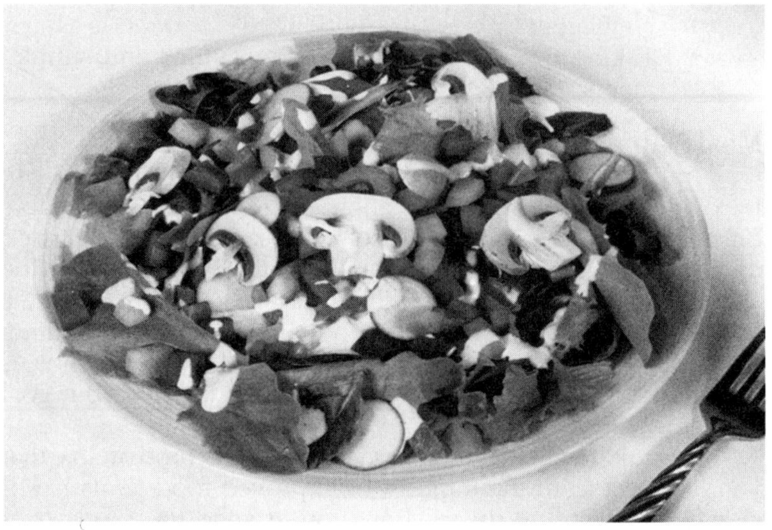

Eating a salad at lunch and supper is a great way to fill up on healthful vegetables.

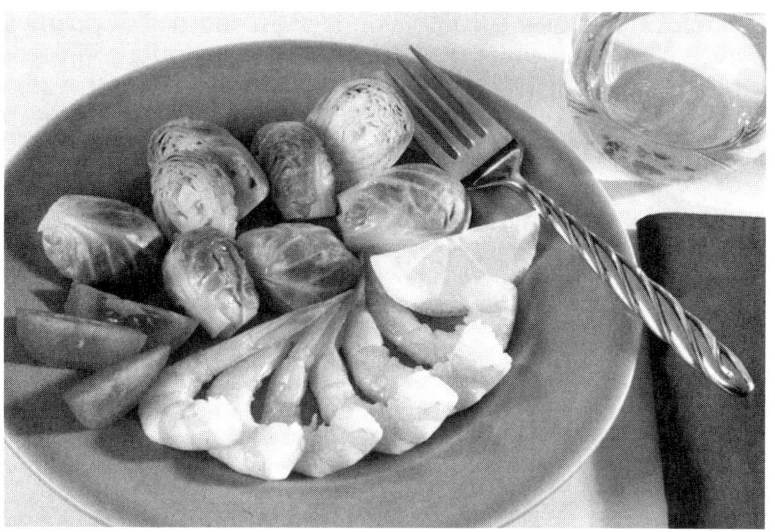

Shrimp is an enjoyable low-calorie choice from the list of approved meats.

Mid-Morning Snack:

1 cup of sliced fresh strawberries sprinkled with Splenda. Beverage: a bottle of zero-calorie Sobe water.

Lunch:

2 cups of romaine lettuce, topped with 1 cup of diced raw vegetables (tomatoes, mushrooms, bell peppers, and radishes), Walden Farms salad dressing, and white chicken breast prepared at home (3 ounces measured before cooking, then diced, season to taste, and cook) Beverage: a tall glass of water.

Afternoon Snack:

80-calorie cup of blueberry Greek yogurt. Beverage: 1 can of Coke Zero.

Late-Afternoon Snack:

Celery sticks. Beverages: a tall glass of water and black tea.

Supper:

Snack on a dill pickle while preparing your salad. 2 cups of iceberg lettuce topped with 1 cup of diced vegetables (tomatoes, cucumbers, radishes, and bell peppers) and calorie-free white wine-flavored vinegar and a sprinkle of seasoning. Pan-fry a 3-ounce patty of 97 percent lean ground beef, season with salt and pepper, top with mustard, and placed on ½ of an open-face Bagel Thin. 1½ cups of fresh vegetables (onions, green beans, squash, and zucchini) pan-fried, seasoned, and served as a vegetable side dish to the open-faced burger. Beverages: a tall glass of water and black decaf coffee.

Evening Snack:

One full-size pink grapefruit, cut in half and baked in the oven with a sprinkle of cinnamon and served with Truvia sweetener. Both grapefruit halves are eaten warm out of the oven. Beverage: a tall glass of water.

Example 2: Daily Meal Plan

Breakfast:

1 cup of 80-calorie fruit-flavored yogurt. Beverage: a tall glass of water and coffee with 1 tablespoon of almond milk (30 calories/cup).

Mid-Morning Snack:

3 pieces of Melba toast with sugar-free jam. Beverage: calorie-free iced tea.

Lunch:

3½ ounces of precooked shrimp with 2 cups of leaf lettuce, fresh lemon juice squeezed over lettuce and shrimp, seasoned with salt and pepper. 2 cups of raw broccoli and cauliflower dipped into Walden Farms dressing. Beverages: 1 green tea and a tall glass of water.

Afternoon Snack:

1 apple sliced and seasoned with cinnamon. Beverages: 1 can diet Dr. Pepper, tall glass of water.

Late Afternoon Snack:

1 dill pickle. Beverage: coffee with 1 tablespoon of almond milk

Supper:

3 ½ oz of tilapia seasoned to taste, wedge of lemon on the side. 1 cup of peas and 1 cup of carrots (measured

before cooking) steamed in water and served on the side. Beverage: tall glass of water.

Evening Snack:

2 kiwi fruit, 2 pieces of Melba toast. Beverage: Iced tea sweetened with Equal and lemon juice.

(In the example for this day, the 2 tablespoons of almond milk are not counted toward the calories for the day, as they represent a trivial number of calories. It allows the person to enjoy coffee who will not drink it black.)

Example 3: Daily Meal Plan

Breakfast:

1 orange, ½ a thin bun toasted and sprayed with "I Can't Believe it's Not Butter" Spray. Beverages: decaf coffee flavored with cinnamon, tall glass of water

Mid-Morning Snack:

80 calorie fruit-flavored yogurt cup. Beverage: zero calorie carbonated water with fruit flavoring.

Lunch:

2 cups of raw vegetables diced and enjoyed on their own. ½ cup of kidney beans seasoned with a zero calorie hot sauce. Beverage: glass of water.

Mid-Afternoon snack:

1 ½ cups of diced watermelon. Beverage: glass of water

Late-Afternoon snack:

Beverage: Diet cola.

Supper:

3½ ounces of tofu with a green leaf salad. 2 cups of asparagus and squash oven-baked and seasoned to flavor. Beverages: a tall glass of water and Earl Grey tea.

Evening Snack:

2 Alessi Italian sesame breadsticks, celery sticks, 10-calorie cup of artificially sweetened Jell-O. Beverage: a tall glass of water.

These three sample meal plans are only a few possibilities from a huge range of possible food combinations that will work on The OWL Diet plan. The important message is that you will select the foods that you personally like, then combine them throughout the day in approved amounts. You will quickly find that the more organized you are with your food, the easier it will be to follow the plan and the more satisfied you will feel with your snacks and meals. Many successful participants pre-measure food and precook their proteins in advance. If you are going to be away from the house for eight or more hours, you must have food with you to eat during that time.

Dr. Abbott and his staff are truly amazing! They helped me lose weight that I've struggled to lose before coming to them. They're angels in my eyes and helped me achieve so much.
Angela, 28

Keep the correct foods portioned and ready to go from the refrigerator. Let other people living with you know what the containers represent. If you are fortunate enough to have someone living with you do the shopping, measuring, and cooking, then you must be sure that they become entirely familiar with the approved foods and portions.

All too frequently I see people fail on the diet due to:

- Eating the wrong foods
- Not eating throughout the day
- Not eating all of the food that is allowed
- Not weighing the meat before cooking

Many people who fail on the diet have not taken the time to learn the food allowances and portions. All too often, these people are eating the wrong foods. They find out the hard way that modifying the diet does not work. Resist the temptation to add foods that are not on the approved list. Once you are eating in maintenance, you will be able to enjoy an even larger range of food options. But remember that maintenance eating is not dieting.

Limited Exercise

The OWL Diet encourages you to be physically active while you are losing weight. It is safe to continue with mild to moderate exercise. More-active levels of activity (such as running) are not safe. Limiting your exercise is such an important topic that it is detailed in chapter 7. If you are not physically active at this time, then I want you to start walking. Now is not the time to join a gym, but it is time to "get off the couch!"

Part II

The Path to Success

4

Prescribed Medications and Hormones

One of the benefits of working with a health care provider while you are on the The OWL Diet is that you have access to a variety of medications and hormones available only by prescription.

Phentermine

Phentermine is an older medication that has been available for many years. Despite its age, phentermine still plays an important role for many successful dieters. It is taken by mouth in either tablet or capsule form, and must be prescribed by a health care provider where you live. Phentermine is classified as an appetite suppressant, and it works well to suppress hunger and food cravings.

I believe that phentermine also stimulates your metabolism. Metabolism describes the rate at which our body uses and burns calories. We do not fully understand why some people have a slower metabolism than others. Patients often state that they believe their multiple attempts at dieting have somehow damaged their metabolism. This could be true, but we don't know for sure. What I do know is that if you can stimulate your metabolism, then you should have greater success in losing weight.

Phentermine therefore has two useful roles to play on The OWL Diet. Its number-one job is to reduce hunger and food cravings. Its number-two role is to stimulate your metabolism. Phentermine can be started on day one of The OWL Diet, or it can be added along the way. It is also a useful adjunct in patients who have been OWL dieting for a few months, have lost weight, but now seem to have hit a plateau where weight loss has slowed or stalled altogether. Adding phentermine at this point seems to kick the diet back into high gear.

By now you are likely excited to try phentermine. Unfortunately, this drug also carries risks and side effects that I will now describe for you. If you are prescribed phentermine, treat it with the respect and caution that it deserves.

I am very busy, and I tend to be a stress eater. I eat most of my calories in the late afternoon and evening. Even though I am only four weeks into the OWL Diet, I definitely feel more in control. When I eat, it's easy to make the right choice.

Abby, 33

As a stimulant, phentermine can increase heart rate and blood pressure and cause heart palpitations. As such, phentermine is not for everyone. If your blood pressure is elevated, then you should not take phentermine. If your blood pressure increases while on this drug, then it must be discontinued. If you are prone to heart palpitations, your health care provider will advise you to avoid phentermine.

Phentermine is related to amphetamines and may not be combined with other stimulant medications. Many adults already take stimulants for attention deficit disorder (ADD) or attention deficit hyperactivity disorder (ADHD). It is not safe to combine a stimulant taken for attention disorders with phentermine as the risk of side effects is greatly compounded. OWL participants who have a history of substance abuse of any type should also avoid use of phentermine. Health care providers should specifically ask about substance abuse, even if it was not voluntarily reported by the patient in their initial report of medical problems.

Phentermine is a controlled medication in the United States. As a result, prescriptions are typically limited to a one-month supply at a time. Daily use of phentermine for two months should be followed by at least a two-week break from the medication prior to restarting its use.

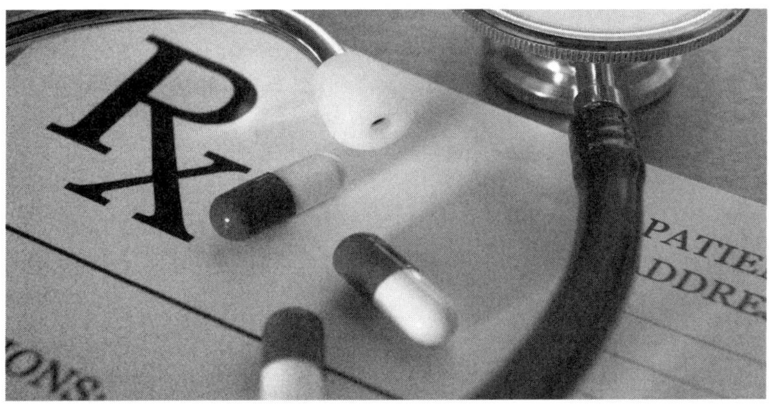

Phentermine and topiramate are both FDA-approved prescription medications that may be used with the OWL Diet.

Phentermine is approved only for active dieting, and should never be used in maintenance (eating better to avoid gaining the weight back). Patients should take care to not lose their supply of phentermine, and should not share it with other people. Phentermine should be stored in a safe location, away from children and anyone who might abuse the drug. Any phentermine that was not used during the diet should be disposed of to avoid accidental use or intentional misuse by other people.

I encourage patients on phentermine to have their blood pressure checked on a weekly basis. If blood pressure increases to an unsafe level, or you report palpitations, then the drug should be discontinued.

Phentermine is typically taken in the morning, with a second dose, if presecribed, at noon, or in the early afternoon. Dosing later in the day is avoided as it may cause insomnia and interfere with sleep.

Your prescribing health care provider will discuss dose options that are available to you. Always follow dosing directions and do not take more medication than is recommended.

Some readers may remember the former popularity of "fen-phen," which was the combination of two prescribed appetite suppressants, one of which was phentermine and the other was fenfluramine. Studies revealed that patients who took fenfluramine were at a higher risk of developing heart valve defects and in 1997 the FDA (Food and Drug Administration) justifiably took fenfluramine off the market, and the drug was no longer available. Phentermine, on the other hand, has never been shown to cause heart valve defects. Belviq is a newer FDA-approved appetite suppressant that is chemically similar to fenfluramine. The concern that Belviq may be associated with heart problems, combined with the slow rate of weight loss seen with this drug, has prevented it from becoming a popular treatment.

Topiramate

Topiramate is an oral medication that is FDA-approved for a variety of conditions, including seizure disorder and to reduce the frequency and severity of chronic migraine headaches. Topiramate may also be prescribed to treat certain mood disorders or chronic pain complaints. Patients who have taken topiramate for these reasons have also reported a side effect of weight loss. How topiramate causes weight loss is not entirely understood. The belief is that topiramate affects how our stomach feels as we are eating.

One of the drives to eat is the perceived need to "fill our stomach" with food. This behavior appears to be more of a bad habit than a real need of the body and can lead to overeating. In North American culture we have been told to "eat all your food" and "clean your plate." In other cultures it is considered a compliment to the chef to leave some food on the plate. (This leaves the impression that you ate so much that you could not finish it all.) In some Asian cultures it is believed that you should stop eating before your stomach feels full. By the time most people feel that their stomach is full, they have actually already eaten too much food.

The effect of topiramate may be that it helps us perceive that our stomach is full after eating a modest amount of food. It may be modifying our drive to keep eating. One thing is clear about topiramate: It is not an appetite suppressant. It does not curb food cravings and hunger the way a stimulant drug such as phentermine can.

When topiramate is used on its own for weight loss the benefit is often minimal. The most common approach is to prescribe topiramate to be taken in conjunction with phentermine. This can be done by prescribing each drug separately or as a combination where the two drugs are combined into one capsule. The combination medication is called "Qsymia."

When I prescribe both phentermine and topiramate for a patient, I prefer to start with phentermine and then add topiramate at a later date, if needed. My goal is to offer a range of treatment options but also recognize that the fewer drugs we need to reach our goal weight, the better. All drugs have potential side effects. By adding one drug at a time, if a side effect does occur it is easier to know which drug to blame. Topiramate also has a long list of potential side effects. A common complaint is drowsiness or loss of mental clarity. For this reason I prefer to dose phentermine in the first half of the day, and topiramate in the second half of the day.

I have lost twenty pounds on The OWL Diet and I am still losing! I have tried many weight loss programs over the years. The support from Dr. Abbott and his staff has helped me be more accountable to myself. Also, I don't get hungry, and I am learning new eating habits.

Ron, 62

Topiramate also carries a specific warning of fetal toxicity. If a woman becomes pregnant while on topiramate, the fetus is at a considerably higher risk of developing a cleft lip or cleft palate abnormality. This toxicity to the fetus occurs very early in pregnancy. By the time a woman realizes that she is pregnant the exposure has likely occurred. Because of the risk to the unborn baby, use of topiramate in women in their reproductive years should be approached with care. Female patients taking topiramate are advised to use a hormonal method (birth control pill) and a barrier method (condoms) of contraception.

Topiramate should not be shared with other people, and unused medication should be disposed of. If you are interested in using topiramate for weight loss you will need to speak in detail with your health care provider about treatment options.

Testosterone

Low testosterone is related to obesity, and using supplemental testosterone may enhance your ability to lose weight. Before I explain how testosterone may help, you need some background information about it.

Testosterone is a hormone that is produced by both men and women. It is beneficial for men and women to have normal levels of testosterone. Testosterone serves important functions in men and women, including the maintenance of muscle mass and a positive effect on energy levels as well as sleep quality.

We also know that testosterone levels are often lower in obese people. When an obese person loses weight, testosterone levels often rebound. Low testosterone has also been blamed for causing deposits of mid-body fat, often referred to as belly fat. It is this very fat, located in the abdomen and hips, that many people older than age forty struggle to lose. Mid-body obesity has also been linked to a higher risk of heart disease and breast cancer. Losing this fat appears to lower that risk.

So now you can see why there is so much interest in testosterone and its relationship to obesity and dieting. Levels of testosterone start dropping after age thirty, and by age forty most men and women have testosterone levels that are below

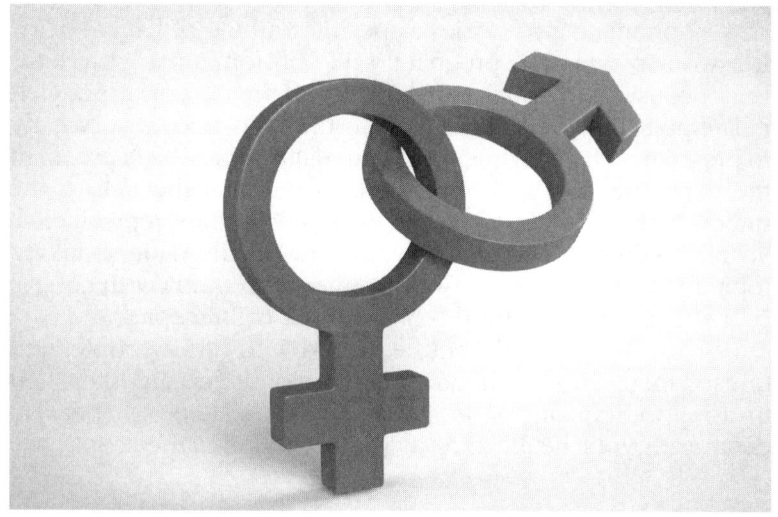

With obesity, testosterone levels are often low in both men and women.

average. Raising testosterone levels in men and women may improve their success at dieting and may be helpful in the battle to lose the mid-body fat bulge.

Enhancing testosterone levels also has several other potentials benefits that may include improvement in energy, less sweating at night, improved quality of sleep, improved emotional well-being, improved mental clarity, improved libido (sex drive), and increased enjoyment of sex (frequency or intensity of climax and orgasm). Improvements in these areas enhance an overall sense of wellness which may in turn improve your rate of success with dieting. If you respond favorably to testosterone, it is a treatment that you could continue indefinitely and may become part of your maintenance plan for keeping weight off.

If you are going to take testosterone, you have several options to choose from. No form of testosterone can be taken by mouth, as it is not absorbed from the stomach. Your choice of testosterone treatments are topical creams and gels, injections into muscle, and the use of testosterone pellets. I will explain each of these options, but first I want to explain the differences between bioidentical and synthetic hormones.

Bioidentical Hormones Compared to Synthetic Hormones

Bioidentical hormones have the same chemical structure as the hormones your body produces. They are an exact copy, an exact match. Your body recognizes bioidentical hormones as having the same structure, and for this reason bioidentical hormones are also often referred to as "natural hormones." Because bioidentical hormones are an exact match to what the body produces, the belief is that they are safer to use.

Synthetic hormones, on the other hand, have a chemical structure that is quite different from natural hormones and do not match what your body produces. Synthetic hormones were developed for human use before bioidentical hormones were developed. One example of synthetic hormone use is birth control pills taken by women to prevent pregnancy.

Synthetic hormones are produced by large pharmaceutical companies that often have a large advertising budget to promote their products to doctors and the public. Bioidentical hormones, on the other hand, are often provided by compounding pharmacies. Compounding pharmacies are able to use drugs and hormones, and on the order of a physician, produce them in unique dosing formats, and even use novel drug delivery systems. The result is that compounding pharmacies are able to produce prescribed treatments that are not available at regular pharmacies. In the United States today, where synthetic hormone prescriptions are regularly written by doctors, the concern has been raised that the use of synthetic hormones may carry a greater risk of side effects.

An example of a synthetic hormone causing problems is the well-documented study showing that women who take the synthetic hormone Premarin are at a higher risk of developing breast cancer. Premarin is a brand name for estrogen derived from the urine of pregnant mares (horses), which likely accounts for how it earned its name (pregnant mares urine). Many women take Premarin after menopause as a source of estrogen replacement therapy.

I lost thirty pounds in two months! I feel wonderful. Through what I learned, I have kept the weight off and know I will be able to continue to do so. I have recommended Dr. Abbott to many of my friends and would never do so if I didn't trust him.

Megan, 36

The oldest method of delivering testosterone for men and women is to give it by injection into muscle. All forms of injectable testosterone are "synthetic," as they have been chemically altered. The bioidentical options for testosterone include the use of sterile pellets and transdermal cream or gels, which are explained below.

Supporters of "natural" bioidentical testosterone therapy believe that synthetic testosterone shots carry greater risk. The bottom line is that we really don't know and probably never will. Why is that? The reason is that multiple forms of testosterone treatments are available, in general use, and accepted as approved treatments.

It costs a great deal of money for large drug companies to perform large clinical trials to try to answer some of the safety questions that arise with the use of hormone prescription treatments. The companies that manufacture these hormones have little incentive to run further studies on products that are already in use. Government funding to pay for such studies is becoming harder to come by. The consumer is left trying to navigate a confusing area where available information about their drugs is inadequate. My belief is that if you are to take supplemental hormones of any type (estrogen, progesterone, testosterone, HCG, and others) then it is best to use bioidentical hormones rather than synthetic ones.

Other Forms of Testosterone: Creams, Gels, and Pellets

As I have said, there is no form of testosterone that can be taken by mouth and be absorbed adequately. What other ways are there to get this hormone into your body? I have already mentioned synthetic injectable testosterone, which is an injection into the buttock that needs to be repeated every one to two weeks on average. Injectable testosterone also has the drawback that, after each injection, your hormone level will be higher, and then drop off steadily until the next dose is given. This fluctuating level of testosterone is less than ideal, as symptoms of low testosterone will also come and go as the hormone levels change.

Two very different delivery systems (the means by which the hormone gets into your body) are available when you choose bioidentical testosterone. When combined with a cream or gel, testosterone can be applied to the skin of the forearm, underarm, thighs, or genital area. The hormone is then absorbed across the skin. Doctors call this method of hormone absorption "transdermal" (meaning "across the skin"). The other bioidentical option is the use of sterile pellets of testosterone that are placed under the skin in the buttock area. To choose between the two options you should consider cost, how well the product raises the level of testosterone, how well it provides a steady blood level of testosterone, and your comfort level in having regular injections.

The problem with all methods of testosterone therapy—topical creams, gels, or injections of testosterone—is what we call the "roller-coaster effect." Levels of testosterone will rise and fall based on when the hormone is applied. Fluctuating levels may cause symptoms to improve only intermittently.

The goal of testosterone therapy is to raise your levels to the upper end of the normal range. Normal levels vary tremendously between men and women. Men often respond positively when their total testosterone blood levels are raised to 1,000. Normal testosterone levels in women are considerably lower, and they respond to modest rises in their testosterone level.

Absorption of hormones across the skin varies between individuals. The biggest challenge with creams and gels is getting the total testosterone to a therapeutic level in men where they may obtain symptom relief. The absorption of testosterone by creams and gels in men is often not adequate.

Dr. Abbott and his staff helped me get my life back! I have been on the diet for almost a month and have lost twenty-two pounds. I've gained my motivation and desire to live again.

Karen, 52

Another concern with testosterone creams and gels is that they must not come in direct contact with the skin of children or pregnant women. An advantage of creams and gels is that the cost may be partially covered by health insurance.

The other form of bioidentical testosterone is the use of pellets that are placed under the skin in the buttock area. The pellets slowly dissolve, releasing testosterone in a slow but continuous manner day and night for three to six months. The benefits of pellets are attainment of excellent blood levels of testosterone, levels that are consistent day and night, and the fact that there is no cream or gel to be applied regularly. Testosterone pellets are inserted during a sterile office procedure performed by a trained individual.

Pellets should not be used in men who want to father children in the future because of the negative effect testosterone supplements may have on fertility (lower sperm count). Women who have a chance of becoming pregnant in the next six months should avoid use of pellets because all testosterone

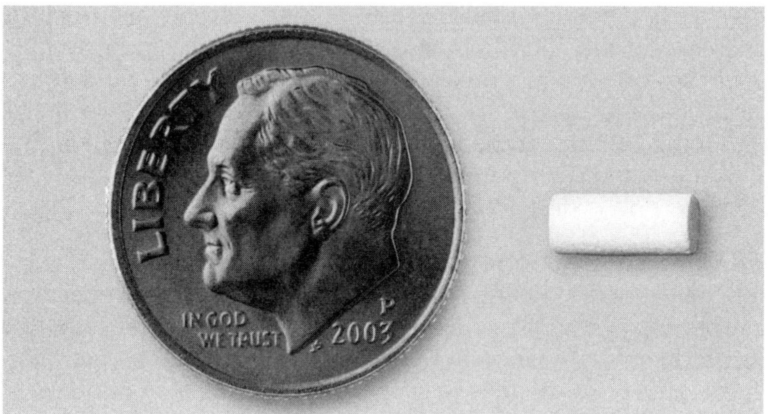

Testosterone, in the form of tiny pellets that are inserted under the skin provide a steady dose of testosterone. One pellet typically lasts for three to six months.

supplements are considered harmful to a fetus and pellets are not typically removed once they are placed, as this is a more involved surgery. Women who are still in their reproductive years should select transdermal creams or gels, as these can be stopped immediately upon discovery of becoming pregnant.

Potential Risks of Testosterone Replacement

One proven risk of using testosterone deserves mention. Testosterone can increase the production of red blood cells in your body. Red blood cells serve the very important function of transporting oxygen to every cell in the human body. If you are low in red blood cells we state that you have anemia. Testosterone has the ability to raise your red blood cells to a level that is considered higher than normal. Having too many red blood cells can increase your risk of blood clots.

If you take testosterone your doctor will measure the number of red blood cells in your body by ordering blood tests on hemoglobin and hematocrit levels. If these tests come back higher than normal, the dose of testosterone will need to be lowered or you will be taken off of testosterone altogether. You may also be required to give up a pint of blood (such as being a blood donor at the Red Cross) to treat the elevated level of red blood cells. Keep in mind that most blood clots occur in people with other risk factors, and elevated red blood cells is only one risk factor.

Other potential side effects of testosterone may include increase in oily skin, increase in acne, increase in body hair, aggressive behavior, breast or nipple tenderness, fluid retention, and increase in the size of the prostate gland (in men). Thinning of hair can be a side effect for men and women, but is not commonly reported by patients as long as the dosing of testosterone is done correctly.

HCG—Human Chorionic Gonadotropin Hormone

As described earlier, human chorionic gonadotropin hormone, more commonly referred to as HCG, is a hormone that is produced by women in huge quantities when they are pregnant. There are theories that if you use a low dose of this hormone, combined with a low-calorie diet, you will lose weight more easily and burn fat more effectively. These theories have never been proven or disproven. Without proof on the effect of HCG in dieting I cannot scientifically claim that there is any benefit. On the other hand, I have an abundance of anecdotal information that HCG may have contributed significantly to the successful weight-loss results achieved in many of my patients. My "biggest loser" was a woman who used HCG, combined with The OWL Diet plan, to successfully lose 140 pounds!

Omaha Med Spa is a fabulous center for weight loss. All employees were very supportive in my journey on The OWL Diet. I've lost twenty-five pounds and have never felt better.

Janelle, 34

What I have observed, unscientifically, is that low-dose HCG also appears to be very safe, and is generally free of any significant adverse side effects. In my medical practice I have had a few people complain of a breakout of acne, and another handful of postmenopausal women report uterine bleeding. In the handful of cases of postmenopausal bleeding, no serious cause of the bleeding (such as cervical or uterine cancer) was found.

There is no proven association between the use of low-dose HCG and a higher risk of any form of cancer, either in men or women. However, in the absence of studies that prove

HCG's safety in women and men with a history of breast cancer, and in men with a history of prostate or testicular cancer, the use of HCG is often avoided in these people.

The FDA and HCG

In the United States, the Food and Drug Administration (FDA) states "HCG has not been demonstrated to be effective adjunctive therapy in the treatment of obesity, there is no substantial evidence that it increases weight loss beyond that resulting from caloric restriction, that it causes a more attractive or normal distribution of fat, or that it decreases the hunger and discomfort associated with a calorie-restricted diet."

In America, the FDA has approved the use of HCG by injection to assist in stimulating ovulation and improving fertility. Because the FDA-approved use of HCG has nothing to do with helping in weight loss, HCG use combined with a low-calorie diet such as The OWL Diet program is an "off-label" use of the prescription hormone. Many drugs in America become FDA-approved for one medical indication and then are reported to be possibly helpful with other conditions. The use of that drug or hormone for a different condition is then considered to be "off-label."

I can report that many OWL Diet participants have faith that HCG has helped them with dieting. I cannot refute or dispute their belief. All forms of HCG used today are bioidentical.

Intramuscular HCG Injections

The FDA stipulates that HCG should be administered by intramuscular injection. *Intramuscular injection* refers to injection of HCG directly into muscle, which results in the best absorption. Self-injection of HCG into the thigh muscle is very easy to learn and can be safely performed at home. HCG should be used only as a prescribed treatment and obtained from a reliable pharmacy.

Patients need to be trained in the proper use of HCG, including:

- Reconstituting HCG by adding the correct amount of sterile bacteriostatic water to a sterile vial containing the correct amount of HCG hormone

- Refrigerating the reconstituted HCG, where it will remain stable for up to sixty days
- Drawing up the correct dose for daily administration
- Correctly injecting the sterile HCG into the thigh muscle

See the Appendix for guidelines on how to give yourself intramuscular injections.

Subcutaneous Injections of HCG: Not Recommended

Subcutaneous injections of HCG refer to injections placed under the skin. These injections are typically self-administered to the fatty layer of the abdomen. I do not support this delivery method as it is not FDA-approved.

HCG has also been used in other forms that are not FDA-approved delivery methods. One form is sold as a liquid drop that is placed under the tongue or swallowed. Absorption by this oral method is likely negligible and its use should be discouraged. The same applies to compounded nasal sprays containing HCG that rely on unproven absorption across the inside lining of the nasal passage.

Topical HCG Cream

HCG may also be prescribed as a topical cream that is applied to the skin for absorption of the hormone across the skin. As mentioned previously, this delivery method is called "transdermal." The use of HCG topical cream is intuitively logical, because we have other FDA-approved transdermal hormone products such as a variety of testosterone creams and gels, and patches used for birth control or to treat menopausal symptoms.

The advantage of transdermal HCG cream is ease of use by simply rubbing it into the skin. Also, it does not need to be refrigerated. The potential disadvantage is that the absorption of hormones varies among individuals using the transdermal method. Some people absorb the hormone better than others. See the Appendix for guidelines on how to use transdermal cream.

HCG and The OWL Diet: Not Recommended during Pregnancy

HCG is the hormone that is looked for when doing blood testing for pregnancy, and in home urine pregnancy testing. Even though a low dose of HCG is used with dieting, it may be detected during pregnancy testing and result in a "false positive" pregnancy test. If a woman believes that she may be pregnant while on The OWL Diet, she must stop the diet, stop the use of HCG, and two days later perform a pregnancy test. If the test is positive at that time, then prenatal care needs to be initiated immediately. Consuming a reduced calorie diet, with the goal of losing weight, is clearly unsafe for a pregnant women and her unborn child.

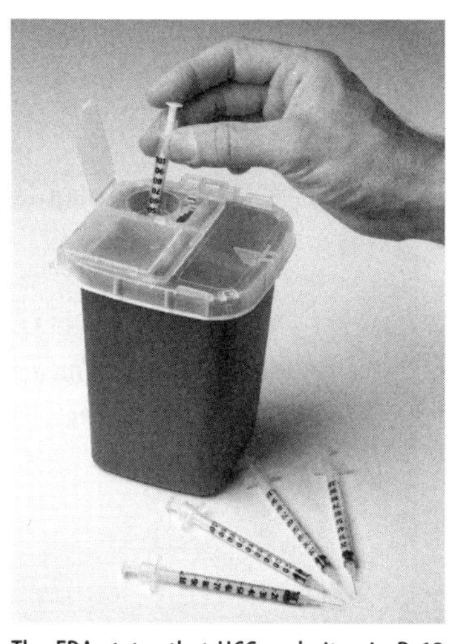

The FDA states that HCG and vitamin B-12 should be injected into muscle. Used needles should be safely disposed, using approved sharps containers.

Low-dose HCG will not on its own increase female fertility, but losing weight may improve a woman's chance of getting pregnant. Low-dose HCG will not interfere with hormonal methods of birth control, such as the birth control pill (oral contraceptive).

Vitamin B-12 Injections

On The OWL Diet I promote the use of supplemental vitamin B-12 in the hope that it will help my patients experience good levels of energy. Vitamin B-12 is also commonly added to multiple vitamin, B-complex vitamins, and "energy drinks" with the same goal of enhancing energy levels. Any claim that the administration of vitamin B-12 is "lipotropic," or helps lose body fat, is false.

Vitamin B-12 is also important for the body to produce red blood cells. Deficiency of vitamin B-12 is called "pernicious anemia." Use of injectable vitamin B-12 is FDA-approved for the treatment of pernicious anemia and the injections are to be administered intramuscularly.

My fiancé and I both needed to lose weight. He was diagnosed with type 2 diabetes in 2007 and has struggled with controlling it. We went on The OWL Diet together. This diet has worked, and together we have lost 150 pounds. My fiancé has been able to control his diabetes without medication.
Ben, 35
Maggie, 28

The use of vitamin B-12 in a person who is not low in B-12 has been found to be entirely safe. Even the use of high doses of vitamin B-12 has not been associated with any harm. The safety profile of vitamin B-12, combined with the desire to have good energy while dieting, makes this vitamin perfect for use on The OWL Diet.

There is another reason that I like additional B-12 use during dieting. Many of my obese patients also suffer from GERD, whereby stomach acid regurgitates into the esophagus, causing symptoms of heartburn. The most common therapy for GERD is one of several medications taken by mouth, collectively known as PPIs (proton pump inhibitors). Examples of PPI medications include Nexium and Prilosec. PPI drugs work very well to suppress the production of stomach acid and alleviate the symptoms of GERD, such as heartburn. However, stomach acid serves a couple of very important functions and patients who are on long-term PPIs may become deficient in vitamin B-12 and are also at a higher risk for pneumonia and certain types of diarrhea.

Losing weight will, in most cases, help reduce the symptoms of GERD, and some patients are able to reduce or discontinue the use of PPI medications. In the meantime, providing supplemental B-12 may help correct any early deficiencies of this important vitamin. For GERD patients, taking vitamin B-12 by injection becomes very important because oral absorption

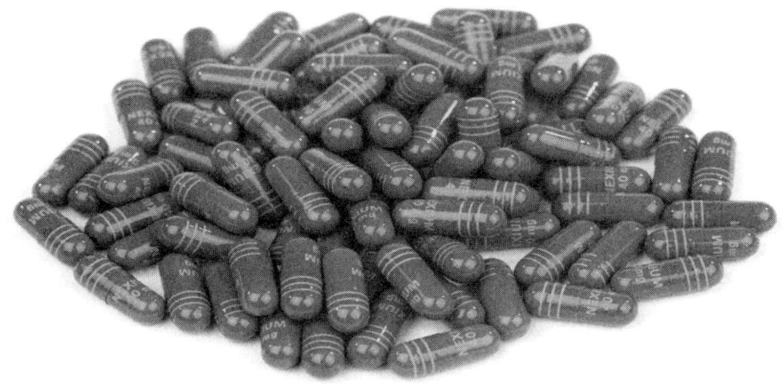

Long-term use of drugs called "proton pump inhibitors," that block acid production in the stomach, have been associated with reduced vitamin B-12 levels.

of B-12 is greatly impaired due to the acid-suppressing effects of the PPI medication that they are taking.

Because HCG and vitamin B-12 are both FDA-approved to be delivered by intramuscular injection, it makes sense to combine them in a single once-daily injection. I have employed this approach for several years, and am pleased with the results and feedback I receive from our patients. If an OWL participant is using transdermal HCG cream, we offer them an injection of vitamin B-12 at each weekly office visit.

5

Vitamins and Supplements

The OWL Diet teaches you to enjoy fresh healthful food. You will be eating generous portions of nutrient-rich vegetables and fruits. The OWL Diet today also provides for the use of low-fat yogurt and low-calorie almond milk, which are excellent sources of calcium. The use of vitamins and supplements is a topic of heated debate in the medical profession. It has been difficult to provide proof through clinical trials that their use is of benefit to our health. Some studies have even claimed taking some supplements can be harmful.

The OWL Diet Pack

I believe that vitamins and supplements can be useful in our diet. I provide OWL dieters with a high-quality dietary supplement that is produced in the United States by a reputable manufacturer. My combination of proprietary ingredients is conveniently packaged and is to be taken with both your lunch and supper. I call my supplements the "OWL Diet Pack." It contains approximately nine calories and may be purchased by anyone in the United States by visiting my Website www.OWLDiet.com.

I have also configured the vitamins and supplements in The OWL Diet Pack so that it can be safely used after you have completed The OWL Diet program, as part of your long-term goal of keeping weight off. This chapter describes the vitamins and supplements I have chosen to use.

Always consult with a physician prior to taking any vitamins or supplements to make sure they are safe for you. Other prescribed therapies may need to be taken at a time that is separate from when you take your dietary supplements.

Garcinia Cambogia (Providing HCA)

Garcinia cambogia is a fruit extract derived from the outer rind of tamarind, a plant that grows in parts of India and other areas in Asia. The active ingredient in this natural product appears to be hydroxycitric acid (HCA). This acid is a derivative of citric acid that is found in a variety of tropical plants, including garcinia cambogia. Small studies have suggested that taking this supplement helps people to lose weight, but the way in which it works remains unknown. This product became popular after it received an endorsement by a popular daytime TV personality. Since then it has become widely available.

The OWL Diet really works! The counseling and friendly staff are all there to help me reach my goal! I feel great!
D.B. woman aged 66

The key to taking garcinia cambogia is finding a reputable supplier, taking the correct dose, and combining its use with a healthful diet plan. The OWL Diet Pack in conjunction with The OWL Diet meets those criteria. You receive a dose of HCA derived from garcinia cambogia in each packet taken with your lunch and supper meals.

Safflower Oil Complex (Providing CLA)

CLA stands for conjugated linoleic acid and in The OWL Diet Pack, it is derived from safflower oil complex. Small studies suggest that CLA may assist with "fat burning" and for this reason I include a dose in each OWL Diet Pack.

Calcium with Vitamin D

I want you to preserve excellent bone health while losing weight on The OWL Diet. To assist you in that, I include a dose of calcium and vitamin D in The OWL Diet Pack. There are many other health benefits of taking both of these supplements if you are deficient in them.

I have selected calcium citrate that yields 250 mg of calcium for use in The OWL Diet Pack. Combined with the calcium that you receive from vegetables such as spinach, broccoli, and Brussels sprouts, along with the calcium in yogurt and almond milk, I believe that you will obtain an adequate total intake of calcium while on The OWL Diet and taking my diet pack.

I also include a generous amount of vitamin D-3 to assist you in achieving optimal health.

Always consult with a physician when you take supplemental calcium or vitamin D, to assure that you are taking the correct amounts. Patients with impaired kidney function, kidney stones, or documented low levels of vitamin D may be directed to alter the dose included in The OWL Diet Pack.

B Complex

Supplemental B vitamins are often promoted for support of adequate energy, the immune system, and mood stability during the menstrual cycle. These claims are not medically substantiated or proven. Nonetheless, many diet participants feel they do benefit from supplemental B vitamins.

I include thiamine (vitamin B-1), riboflavin (vitamin B-2), niacinamide, pyridoxine (vitamin B-6), folic acid, biotin, and vitamin B-12 in my "B-complex" portion of The OWL Diet Pack.

B-complex vitamins can cause nausea if taken without food and are therefore taken at meal time. Your urine will turn a darker orange or yellow color for several hours after each dose.

Always consult with a physician to see if it is recommended for you to take B-complex vitamins.

Fiber-Plex

I include "Fiber-Plex" (proprietary blend produced by Douglas Laboratories) twice a day as part of The OWL Diet Pack. This grain-free blend of fiber is also lactose-free. When taken at mealtime with water, fiber will distend in the stomach and help your stomach to feel full. Fiber also assists bowel function by adding bulk to the stool to help ensure regular normal bowel movements while you are dieting.

Potassium

On 800 calories per day, your body will be burning fat to generate additional calories needed for metabolism. As part of this process, your body produces additional acids. Acids affect the acidity level (pH) in the body. With an increase in acidity, potassium levels shift within the body (acidity drives potassium into cells and away from the bloodstream).

Lower potassium levels may cause muscle weakness or cramping. If potassium levels drop too low, cardiac irregularities may occur (palpitations, irregular heart rate, and arrhythmia). Too much potassium in the body can cause problems as well.

I include a very small dose of potassium in The OWL Diet Pack. The dose is 99 mg as an "over-the-counter" (available without a prescription) source of potassium. I have found that by including this very small dose of potassium I rarely have OWL participants report muscle weakness or cramping.

Always consult with a physician before taking any form of potassium supplements. Not all people should take them. Certain medical conditions such as impaired kidney function will affect potassium levels. Certain medications may raise or lower potassium levels as a drug side effect.

6

Simple Rules of "OWLology"

No, "OWLology" is not a real word. But I hope you'll find it to be a catchy word that you will remember as you are following The OWL Diet plan. I would like for you to think of it as a few simple rules about how we eat and drink on The OWL Diet.

These rules are simple: eat food from the allowed list throughout the day, and drink lots of fluids to stay well hydrated. It's that easy! Try your best to permanently adopt this more healthful way of eating. Think of it as if you're making it a "part of your DNA."

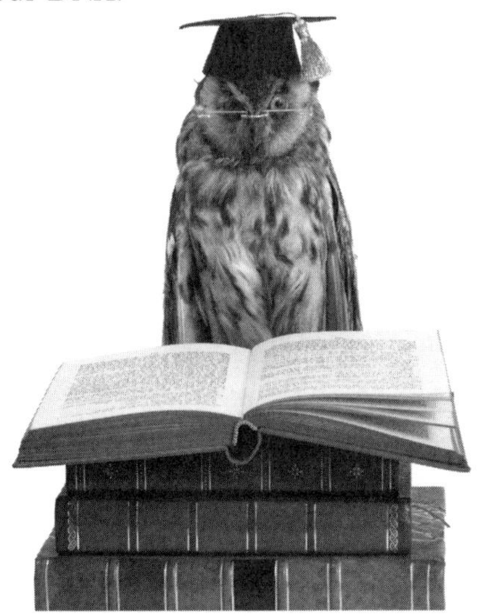

OWLology is learning to eat food throughout the day and to stay well hydrated.

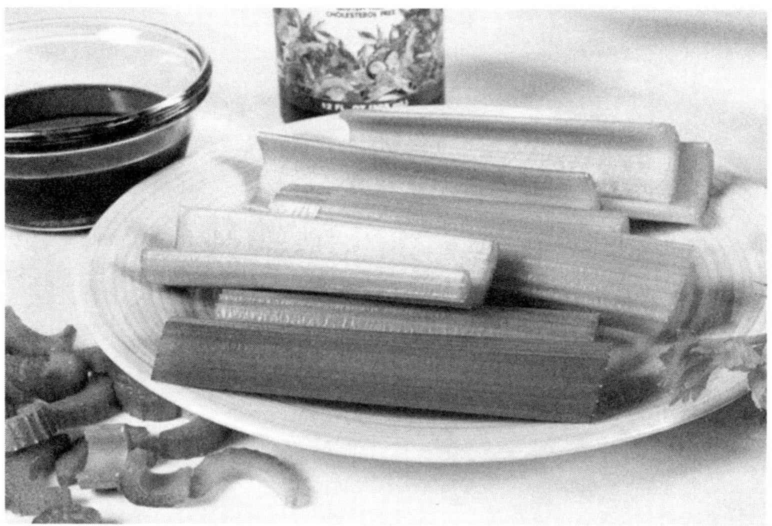

Celery is considered a "free" food, meaning you can eat unlimited amounts of it.

Three Meals a Day

How many times have you heard the expression, "You should always eat three meals a day"? It turns out the experts are right—you should eat at least three meals per day. If you skip meals, you'll likely develop a slower metabolism, so you eat less but don't lose weight! Yet, many people skip meals. The list of excuses is long and includes:

- I don't have time to eat breakfast in the morning.
- I am not hungry when I get up.
- I have a snack in the car on the way to work.
- They don't give us enough time at lunch to eat a real meal.
- Everyone brings snacks to work, and I eat them all day long.
- I don't like cooking or I don't know how to cook.
- I skip lunch so I can eat more at suppertime.
- I am trying to cut back so I can lose weight.
- I go right to the gym after work, so I don't have time for supper.

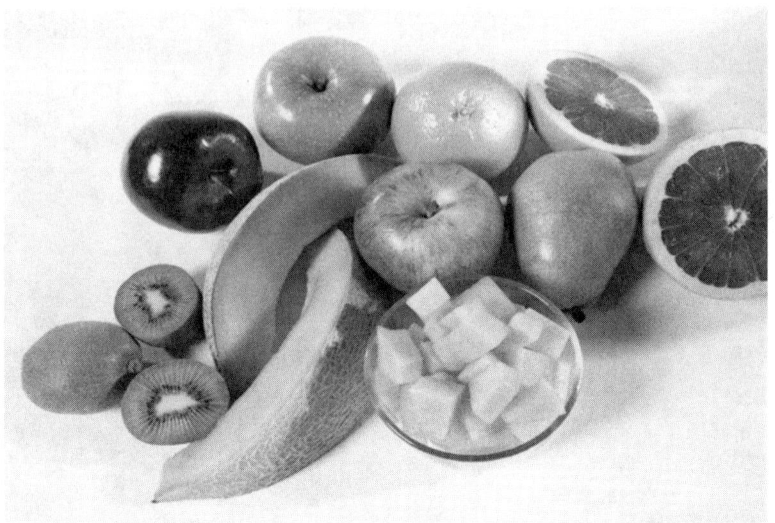

Fresh fruit makes a good snack. You are allowed three fresh fruits daily. Check the list of fruits you may choose from on page 90.

- My kids have activities after school, so we don't have time to prepare and eat a proper dinner.

Do any of these excuses sound familiar?

Eating breakfast in the morning stimulates your metabolism and contributes to better energy during the day. Learning and memory are also enhanced by eating proper meals.

The OWL Diet insists that you have three meals per day. I call them breakfast, lunch, and supper—but you can call them whatever you want. You must learn to follow this eating pattern while dieting, and you should continue this healthful eating habit for the rest of your life!

Three Snacks a Day

When I tell participants that they will have three meals and three snacks per day on a total of about 800 calories per day, many people are surprised. Snacking alleviates hunger and food cravings. By adding three small snacks per day you will be "grazing" on and off all day long. You will also always have a small snack to look forward to!

Common snacks include a serving of fruit or yogurt, but may also include raw vegetables or a portion of your bread allowance for the day. Calorie-free snacks include celery and dill pickles.

Water, Water, Water

Studies have shown that an adequate intake of water is associated with weight loss. Drinking enough water is not just important to success with dieting, but is also a key component of health and wellness. It is surprising how many people do not drink enough water over the course of every day. Water is the source of life! Most of our body is water! Many people in underdeveloped countries wish they had access to more clean water, but most of us take it for granted.

On The OWL Diet you will be using water to burn fat. Water keeps your metabolism (the rate that you burn calories) stimulated. Adequate water intake ensures that you are hydrated and less likely to feel weak, dizzy, or light-headed. Dehydration leads to low blood pressure that could cause you to faint and hurt yourself. Drinking an adequate amount of water may also reduce your urge to consume beverages that contain sugar and calories.

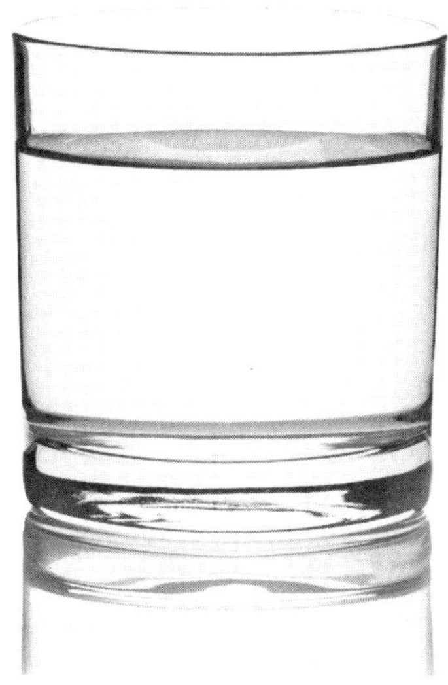

Water is essential in burning fat. Drink at least eight, 8-ounce glasses (one-half gallon) of water daily. If you prefer, drink flavored waters that have zero calories in them.

How much water do we need? I believe that a minimum is half gallon per day, and a full gallon per day is better. In metric terms think of two to four liters of water per day. Spread it out over the course of the day. Inadequate amounts of water can raise your risk for kidney stones, impaired kidney function, constipation, aging skin, fatigue, and muscle cramps. Some common reasons I hear from people who don't drink enough water include:

- I don't like the taste of water.
- I forget to drink water.
- I don't have time to drink water.
- I don't want to have to go to the bathroom more often.
- It is hard at work for me to get to a bathroom.
- I don't want to have to get up at night to urinate.
- When I drink more water I don't always make it to the bathroom in time.

None of these are an acceptable excuse for not drinking enough water. Make it a point to drink enough water on The OWL Diet, and maintain that healthful habit for the rest of your life.

Using Artificial Sweeteners, Carbonated Water, and Caffeine

If you struggle with drinking enough water, try flavored beverages that are carbonated and calorie-free. There are now many brands of artificial sweeteners available. They are all calorie-free, so any of them can be used while losing weight on The OWL Diet.

Carbonated water is also calorie-free and may be counted towards your water intake. Caffeine is allowed on The OWL Diet. Caffeine is found in many beverages such as soda pop, coffee, tea, and some energy drinks. Caffeine is a diuretic—it stimulates the kidneys to produce more urine. While you are allowed caffeinated beverages, you still need to drink an adequate amount of water as well. Beverages that contain caffeine do not count toward your water intake for the day.

If you wish to reduce your caffeine intake, I suggest you do so gradually. Stopping caffeine altogether may cause withdrawal headaches and strong cravings for it.

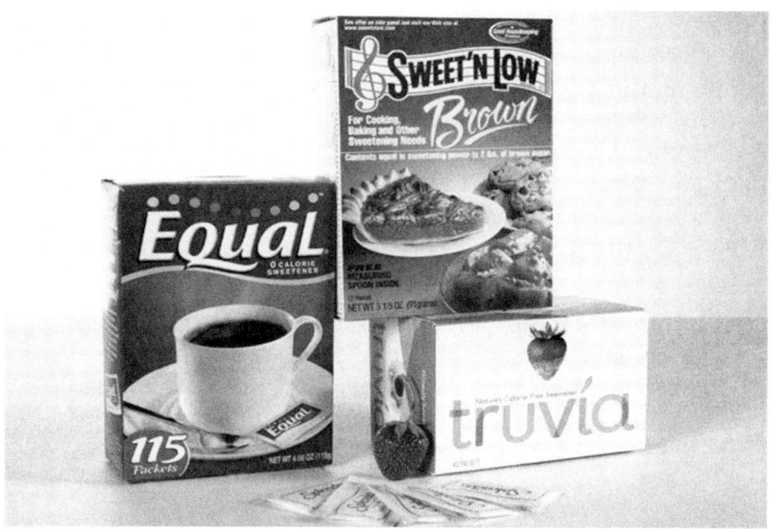

You may use any of the sugar-free sweeteners that are available today. Make sure they contain no sugar or carbohydrates, which turn into sugar once ingested.

Measure and Weigh Food Portions

A common cause of failing to lose weight, or losing weight slower than expected, is that people don't measure and weigh portions. The OWL Diet is very specific about quantities. Guessing is not measuring. Estimating weight based on "the size of a deck of cards" or "the size of the palm of your hand" is not a good plan.

Chicken, beef, turkey, seafood, and other sources of meat must be weighed before cooking because that is how dieticians calculate the calories in meats. When meat is cooked, water may be removed during the process, making an ounce of cooked meat higher in calories than before cooking. One exception I make to this rule on The OWL Diet is a once-a-day allowance of 7 ounces of shrimp that have been precooked by steaming them (until pink) with water. Because no oil is used in cooking shrimp this way, the calories of the cooked shrimp compared to raw shrimp are very similar. Cooked shrimp is sold in packages with a set weight and labeled calorie count.

Another cause of failure on the diet is that some OWL dieters have misjudged the daily allowance of vegetables, which is stated as a total of four cups of fresh *uncooked* vegetables per day, choosing no more than one cup of any particular vegetable—and you are not allowed to have corn. One gentleman insisted that he was following the diet, but he was not losing weight quickly enough. Upon further questioning, it turned out he was eating four cups of *cooked* squash every day, and was breaking two key rules: He was choosing one vegetable instead of a minimum of four different ones, and he was measuring the vegetable cooked rather than uncooked.

I gained twenty-five pounds while dating my future husband, another twenty-five while pregnant with our child, and another twenty-five as a new mother. I dieted for the next twenty-two years without success. Then, I found Dr. Abbott's program. I have lost sixty-five pounds and plan to shed the final ten this month!

Anne, 53

I also specify on the diet that up to four cups of fresh lettuce greens, divided per day into two salads, is considered "free." One woman some years ago was crying at her first-week weigh-in visit because she had not lost any weight, but believed she was following the diet. In turns out she had eaten large quantities of frozen *cooked* spinach. As a salad, green spinach is certainly allowed, but four cups of *fresh* spinach will cook down to a very small amount. She had been heating and eating two large frozen blocks of cooked spinach every day!

To avoid confusion on food choices and measurements, I train my staff to quiz diet participants with specific food enquiries every week. We are not looking to find a "cheater." We are trying to help dieters avoid making common innocent errors in labeling and measuring.

I suggest that you learn the approved OWL Diet food choices and measurements inside and out, and your meal planning will become second nature.

If you have a two-week period of time in which you have lost no weight, it may be a good time to review the diet guidelines again so you can analyze the foods you have eaten. Chances are that you will find the problem, make the adjustments, and get back on track with losing weight.

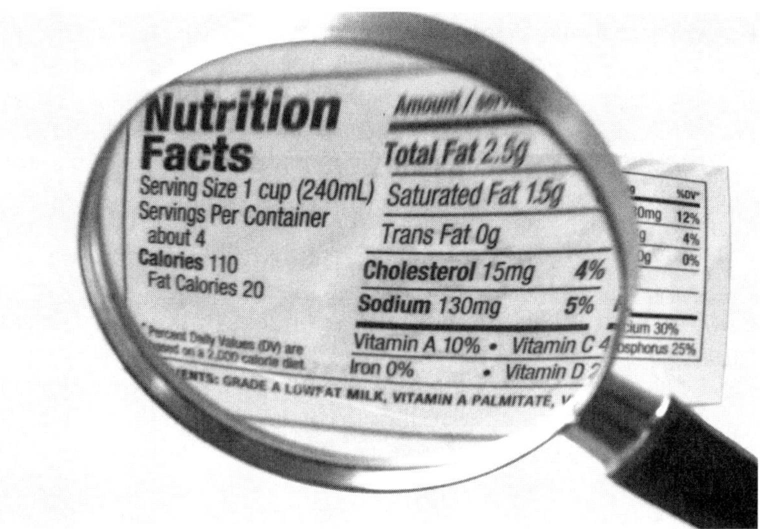
Nutrition
Facts
Serving Size 1 cup (240mL)
Servings Per Container
about 4
Calories 110
Fat Calories 20
Total Fat 2.5g
Saturated Fat 1.5g
Trans Fat 0g
Cholesterol 15mg 4%
Sodium 130mg 5%
Vitamin A 10% • Vitamin C
Iron 0% • Vitamin D
GRADE A LOWFAT MILK, VITAMIN A PALMITATE,

Learning to read food labels is important. Note serving sizes and calories per serving.

Read Food Labels Carefully

Another common error that we have all made is to read the "calories per serving" and "serving size" incorrectly. Labeling can be very misleading. A container of yogurt may appear compliant with a label of "80 calories per serving," only you find out later that there are two servings per container.

When it comes to flavored beverages the label must state "calories per serving: zero." Many diet beverages, diet tea for example, have calories.

Many people are tricked into thinking that any product labeled as "diet," "sugar-free," or "fat-free" will surely work on The OWL Diet. The truth can be quite the opposite because many items labeled as fat-free are not calorie-free. There have been many times I read the total calories in a dessert or bag of chips and been shocked into putting it back on the shelf! Be careful, and become a good label reader.

Once you have mastered the habit of reading labels carefully, it will serve you well not just as you're dieting but also in maintaining your weight loss.

Counting Calories not Required

Most of the people participating in my diet plan state, "I have done all the other diets already." Often, they have counted calories in the past, and are relieved to know they do not have to count calories on The OWL Diet. I have already made the calorie calculations for each food item, but they are approximated.

On the other hand, you want to count calories, you are certainly welcome to do so. Some people enjoy this part of dieting, and it helps them to stay on track. In the era of smart phones and apps that count calories, there are certainly people who enjoy calorie counting. Kudos to them! I have seen detailed Excel flowcharts detailing food choices made and calories consumed, but you need to know this is not expected of you!

The reality is that the calorie count of a measure of food will vary depending on the source you use to calculate calories because different books and "apps" vary from one another. Furthermore, the size of some food items will vary. For example, the size of an apple or orange can vary by a large amount, and so will its calories.

On average, if you were to count calories, you would find that, most days, my diet adds up to approximately 800 calories per day.

I never want you to get below 600 calories per day, and if you have a particularly physical job then we may advise you to increase your intake to 1,000 calories or more per day.

The OWL Diet is based on selecting the foods that are allowed, in the correct portions, spread out over the course of the day. If you follow the plan, it will work for you. We don't need to make it more difficult than it needs to be.

7

Exercise Dos and Don'ts

It is important to fully understand the role that mild to moderate exercise plays while you are on The OWL Diet program. I prefer to use the expression "physical activity" instead of "exercise." The word "exercise" may sound intimidating to a person who is overweight. Few things in life are more threatening for many overweight people than the thought of being in a gym surrounded by people who have bodies perfectly sculpted from years of working out.

The thought of squeezing your body into a pair of tight shorts and facing yourself in the mirror may make you shudder when the topic of exercise is raised. Aside from disliking our own body image, the realities of exercise may seem painful—sweating, shortness of breath, muscle cramps, and debilitating fatigue the next day. With this in mind, "physical activity"sounds more achievable than the word "exercise."

Physical activity is a vital component of good health. Regular fitness has been shown to reduce the risk for heart disease, strengthen bones, maintain joint flexibility, and manage blood pressure as well as blood sugar (to mention just a few benefits). I'm most certainly a proponent of being physically active at all stages of life. The good news is that you do not have to work out *hard* to achieve the health benefits of exercise. Mild to moderate forms of exercise such as walking, stretching, pool aerobics, and outdoor yard work are excellent forms of activity, and all work well on The OWL Diet plan.

You may even be getting enough physical activity while you are working. Examples include electricians, plumbers, and

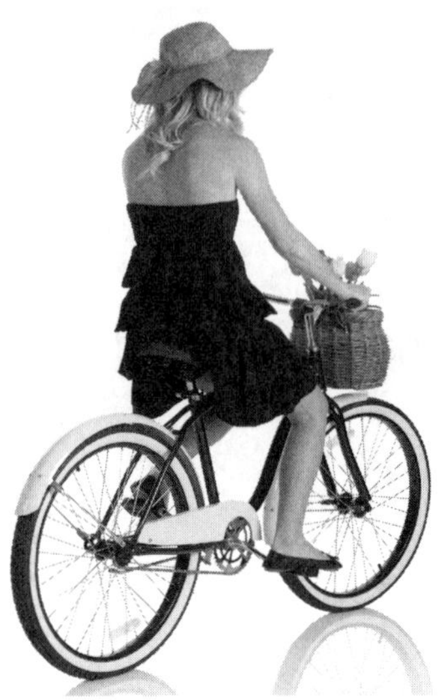

Because The OWL Diet is a low-calorie food plan, strenuous exercise is not advised. However, an exercise such as moderate walking and bicycling is allowed.

construction workers. If your job has you standing or walking most of your workday, then you are getting exercise. Add to this the continual movement of the arms that occurs in many jobs such as assembly work, stocking, shipping, or working as a cashier. The list goes on and on.

If, on the other hand, you commute to work by car or public transit and then spend most of the day sitting at a desk, then your job is very sedentary and your physical activity level needs to be increased away from your job.

Now is a good time to assess the amount of physical activity you get daily. Do you walk or ride a bicycle to work? Once you are at work, are you standing, walking, or climbing stairs? Do you lift boxes or heavy items? If you get personal time during the day for lunch and breaks, how do you spend that time?

At home, are you climbing stairs, doing laundry, cleaning the house, running after small children, gardening, cleaning the yard, or walking the dog? You may be getting more physical activity than you realize. Also assess your level of recreational activity. Do you walk the golf course or use a power cart? Are you participating in classes such as yoga, dance, or aerobics?

Exercise Dos

The low-calorie diet that you will follow on The OWL Diet plan will provide you with the energy you need to perform day-to-day activities. You are also encouraged to be physically active in a mild to moderate way.

When you are on The OWL Diet, *I do allow* the following mild to moderate physical activities:

- Household activities such as laundry, cleaning, and yard work
- Going to the gym or exercising at home—thirty minutes of light yoga, spinning, stretching, walking, swimming, or light weights (no more than ten pounds per hand)

Exercise Don'ts

When you are on The OWL Diet, I ask that you not exercise to the point that:

- Your heart rate increases to over 120
- You are breathing hard
- You are sweating heavily

Examples of exercise that is not permitted include:

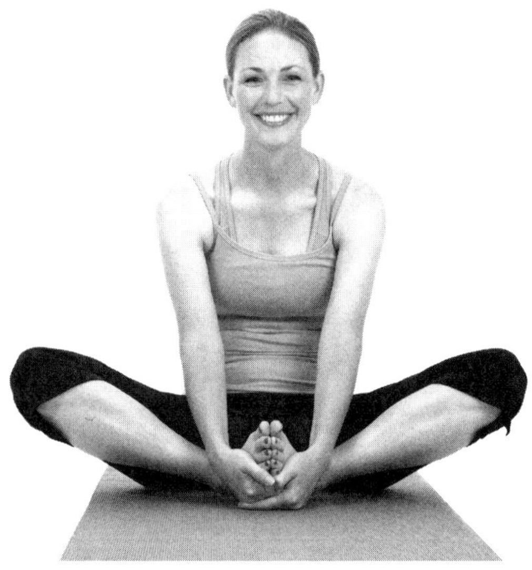

Yoga is an approved activity as long as you stay well hydrated.

- Running
- Walking over 3.5 mph, especially on an incline
- Pushing hard on a bicycle ride
- Swimming lengths of the pool
- Weight lifting over twenty pounds

You cannot train for a half marathon and start The OWL Diet! If you were to try to do so, you would become weak and light-headed and you might faint. You might even develop an irregularity of your heart beat called an arrhythmia. On any diet where you are losing an average of three to four pounds per week the body is burning fat very quickly. One result of that fat burn is the production of acids, a condition called "ketoacidosis." With ketoacidosis the pH level in your body is lower (the acidity is higher) and potassium will shift from outside of cells to inside of them. Drops in potassium can affect your heart and muscles, and problems can occur from too much activity.

When determining if a particular activity is safe on The OWL Diet, keep a few basic rules in mind: If your heart rate is over 120 or you are sweating or breathing hard during that activity, then don't do it! You are placing yourself at risk of causing harm. Weight loss needs to be done in a safe fashion,

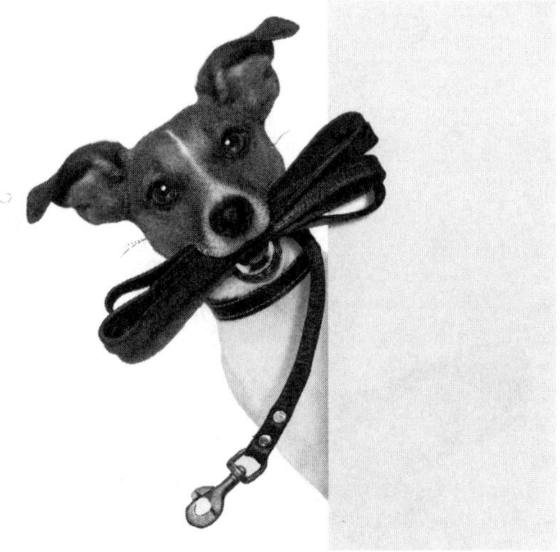

Walking the dog for fifteen to thirty minutes is good for both of you!

with the goal of improving your health, not increasing your risk of developing a problem.

Do not undertake new activities that were not a part of your routine prior to starting The OWL Diet. When in doubt, it is always best to consult your physician.

If, during the course of day-to-day activities, you feel light-headed, weak, or dizzy, then take a break and consume additional water as well as foods that are approved on The OWL Diet. If you continue to not feel well, then contact your doctor or seek immediate medical attention.

After seeing the success my wife had on The OWL Diet, I decided to try it, too. I lost fifty pounds in four months. The staff was very supportive during my weight loss. I would highly recommend this diet to anyone interested in losing weight.

Martin, 50

Some patients who insist on continuing strenuous physical activity invariably fail on The OWL Diet. Even when they have been told to cut back on their exercise, they often hide it from the health care provider who is monitoring them on the diet. The reason given for engaging in unapproved levels of physical activity is the false hope of accelerating the rate of weight loss. Why does this approach fail? The reason is simple. Excessive exercise combined with low-calorie dieting is not only dangerous, it also leads to tremendous hunger cravings. The ravenous hunger that is created by high levels of exercise cannot be suppressed, and inevitably leads to an increased intake of food and calories. Those additional calories are frequently greater than the calories burned off during the activity, and your rate of weight loss slows.

Other dieters who do not heed my warnings about strenuous exercise and continue against medical advice do so for a different reason. They crave the high level of physical exercise that they are accustomed to. Part of this drive is the positive endorphin hormone release that occurs with exercise. Endorphins make us feel better by alleviating feelings of stress or anxiety. Runners who are forced to stop running due to ill-

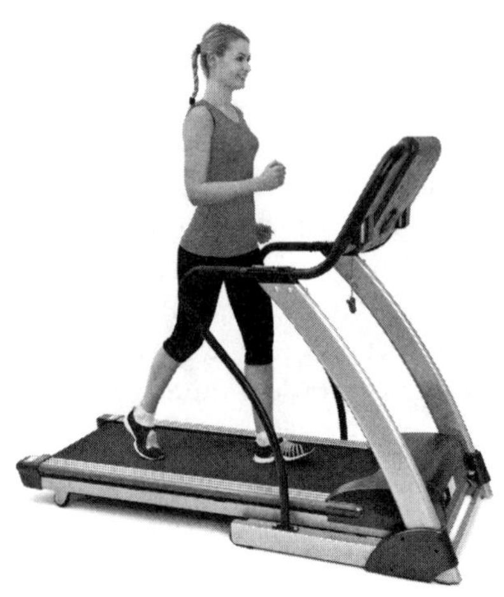

Walking on a treadmill for thirty minutes, at a speed of up to 3.4 miles per hour, is the top end of what is allowed.

ness may experience endorphin withdrawal that can lead to depressed moods.

Another reason some people exercise too much, despite my warnings, is their fear that a reduction of physical activity will lead to a reduction in muscle mass, strength, and muscular appearance of their body. It is true that reduced exercise of muscle groups will lead to reduced muscle mass, but the degree to which this occurs over one or two months of OWL dieting is minimal.

In men or women prior to age forty, muscle has tremendous memory and muscle strength and mass is quickly restored by increasing activity, but only after completion of The OWL Diet. After the age of forty, assessment of testosterone levels may play an integral part in maintenance of muscle mass during and after dieting. As discussed in chapter 4, testosterone levels below the median are easily raised with bioidentical testosterone with the goal of maintaining muscle mass and promoting loss of mid-body fat.

When you complete The OWL Diet and you've reached your goal weight, you can then engage in more physical activity. In fact, I think you will find it will be much more enjoyable to do so because of your lower weight. Regular physical exercise is an excellent way for you to *maintain* the weight you've lost.

What If I Can't Exercise at All?

Some OWL dieters cannot engage in even mild physical activity due to current health problems. Some examples are:

- Severe arthritis limits walking to only 100 feet at a time, and only with use of a walker.
- Multiple sclerosis limits a person's walking to only within a small apartment, with use of a cane. Trips outside the home are only possible with use of a power scooter.
- Parkinson's disease causes tremors with the result that walking is limited to short distances and only with personal assistance to prevent falls.

If your mobility is limited due to a medical condition, on The OWL Diet plan we will ask you to be as active as is reasonable and safe for you. Even doing a small amount of activity will help stimulate your metabolism and help you to feel better. Many health problems that limit mobility have also contributed to that individual gaining weight in the first place.

The good news is that these people will still lose weight by following the low-calorie diet as described in this book. Weight loss will be slower, but is still achievable. Some patients in this group may need to reduce calorie intake to the minimum

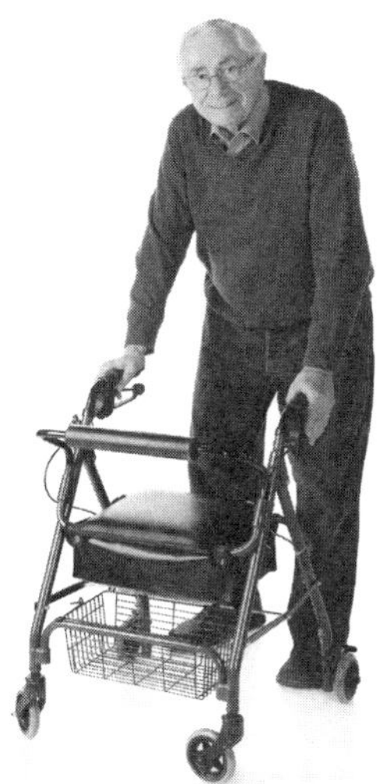

With reduced mobility you will still lose weight on The OWL Diet.

of 600 calories per day that is allowed on The OWL Diet. One of the best ways to reduce calories is the elimination of the 100 calories per day that is otherwise allowed from the "bread and grain" category.

Part III
The OWL Diet Food Plan

8

Approved Foods and Beverages on The OWL Diet

It is important that you become completely familiar with what foods are allowed on The OWL Diet. Part Three of this book is your reference guide, and you will want to come back to it frequently during your weight-loss journey.

Read this part of my book with great care. Not all of the food mentioned will interest you. Your goal is to select the foods that you prefer, and then determine how you will divide them during the course of the day. The OWL Diet encourages you to have three meals per day—I call them breakfast, lunch, and supper. You should also plan on three snacks per day, taken between the three meals. Choose the beverages that you will use. Make sure you get enough water over the course of the day to stay well hydrated.

Beverages

The most important message here is to drink lots of water. I tell my patients, "Drink water for weight loss and drink water for life." I want you to keep drinking adequate amounts of water from this day forward.

Water: Eight Glasses a Day

Water is important for the following reasons:

- Water is consumed by the body during the course of metabolism, and your body will be very busy converting body fat to energy.
- Water helps to curb your appetite and to maintain your energy.

- Water allows your kidneys to filter blood and generate an efficient output of urine.
- Water will reduce your risks of headaches and dizziness.
- Water helps you have regular bowel movements.

You may drink water from many different sources, including tap water, filtered water, carbonated water, and bottled water.

Some people struggle with consuming enough water every day. They find it helpful to drink flavored beverages that are calorie-free and caffeine-free and count them as part of their daily water intake. These flavored drinks often contain artificial sweeteners and may be carbonated. When deciding if a beverage is approved on the diet plan, you must read the label for "calories per serving" and confirm that it states *zero* calories.

There are two types of calorie-free beverages that are allowed on The OWL Diet, but they do not count toward your water intake. They are soda pop and caffeine-containing fluids.

Soda Pop and Soft Drinks

Depending on where you live you may be using the term "soda," "pop," or "soft drinks" to refer to the category of beverages that I call "soda pop." These beverages are all carbonated and come in a wide variety of flavors. All soda pops are sweet, which likely is what makes them very appealing to many of us. The sweetness is derived from sugar, high fructose corn syrup, natural sweeteners such as Stevia, or artificial sweeteners. The choice of sugar or sweetener determines whether a soda pop is "diet" or "regular." Diet soda is calorie-free and regular soda is quite high in calories. Some soda contains caffeine, while others are caffeine-free.

Soda pop occupies a large amount of space in most grocery stores, supermarkets, and gas stations. We are exposed to a lot of advertising promoting soda. Many people consume soda pop throughout the day, even at breakfast. Some people consume more soda pop per day than water.

Soda pop comes in many different sizes and forms—from cans and bottles to plastic containers and in large cups at soda fountains. Many consumers have a preference for one flavor or another, such as cola versus fruit flavoring. My overwhelming

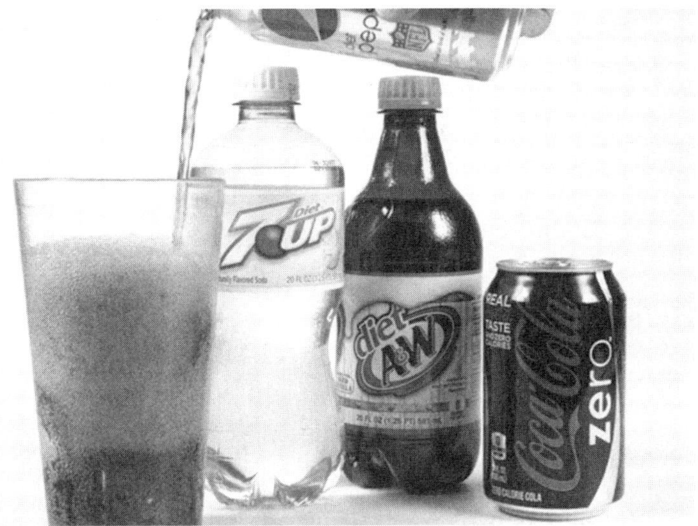

Diet pop, although not healthful for you, is allowed on The OWL Diet, but does not count toward your water intake.

observation has been that people in general love the taste of soda pop, and it can become very habit forming.

Soda pop is not a healthful beverage for the following reasons:

- It has no nutritional value—there is nothing in it that is good for us.
- It has a high phosphate content, which interferes with calcium absorption into bone and may raise the risk for osteoporosis.
- It has a high salt content.

It may fuel, rather than satisfy, our cravings for other sweet foods. Despite all of these negative facts about soda pop, the reality persists that many people will want to continue soda while they diet and for the rest of their life.

My goal is to help you lose weight. Toward that goal, you may be pleased to know that I allow diet soda pop on The OWL Diet, but here are the rules:

- Limit your consumption to no more than 8 fluid ounces per day. That equates to one can or one small plastic bottle per day.

- Your soda pop must be diet and it must be calorie-free.
- It may contain caffeine.
- Soda pop consumption does not count toward your water intake for each day, even if it is caffeine-free.
- There is no "exchange" allowed with soda pop—you either choose to have it or lose it each day, but you cannot exchange it for another food.

Caffeinated Drinks

Caffeine is added to many beverages, due to its stimulant effects. Many of us become reliant on our caffeine for a variety of reasons, such as:

- It gets us up and going in the morning with a boost of energy.
- It wakes us up and improves mental alertness.
- It fights the effects of feeling sleepy or drowsy during the day.
- It can stimulate our bowels to move.

Caffeine has other effects that I consider undesirable, such as:

- It acts as a "diuretic" to stimulate an increased production of urine that in turn may lead to dehydration.
- It has addictive tendencies so we crave our next caffeine fix.
- Stopping caffeine often leads to withdrawal headaches.
- It may increase heart rate and cause palpitations.
- It can make us feel more anxious or nervous.

Caffeine is unique in its relationship as to how it affects our appetite for food. This effect varies among people. It may increase hunger, reduce hunger, or have no effect on hunger at all. What effect does caffeine have on you?

When I take all of the above factors into consideration, it's clear to me that caffeine is a drug. Some of us are able to use caffeine safely and in ways that we find beneficial. Others are better off to avoid caffeine altogether.

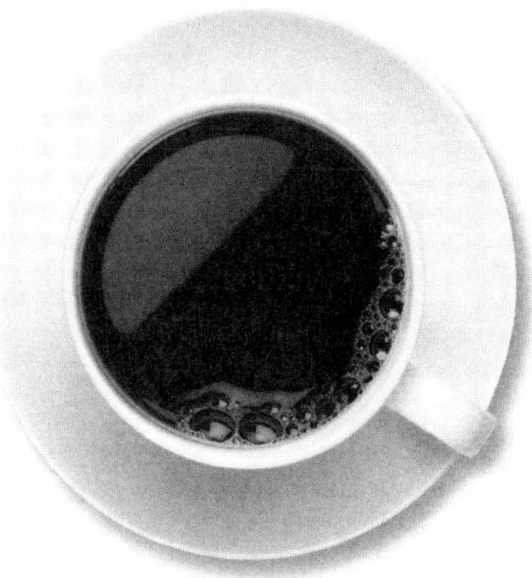

Drink your coffee black, or use a small amount of low-calorie almond milk or zero-calorie artificial sweeteners.

On The OWL Diet, I allow the use of caffeine. Keep in mind that caffeine is found in coffee, tea, soda pops, and energy drinks. Remember that these caffeine-containing drinks must be calorie-free and they do not count toward your daily water intake.

Milk

Cow's milk, that is, is not allowed on The OWL Diet. Here is my reason: It is too high in calories! When I was selecting beverages for The OWL Diet, I explored this option, because I enjoy milk and dairy products, as do many of my patients. When I was at my personal maximum weight I was consuming the following dairy products on a regular basis: butter, cheese, ice cream, and 1 percent milk. It surprised me to find how many calories were in these foods.

I turned to skim milk. I said to myself, "Surely, fat-free milk would work on this diet." Again I was shocked by what I found: Even fat-free (skim) milk was a whopping eighty calories per cup. Cow's milk was clearly not going to work on my diet plan.

Nondairy creamers are not calorie-free and are not allowed on my diet. Fat-free creamers fall into the same category; although they are fat-free, they are still too high in calories.

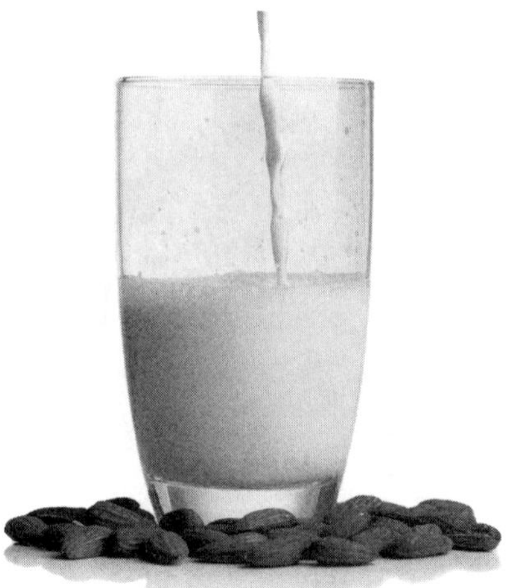

Nuts are not allowed while dieting, but low-calorie almond milk may be used in moderation.

I am not stating that dairy products are unhealthful or bad for you. In fact, they are an excellent source of calcium. My opinion is that the calorie allowance on The OWL Diet is better spent on consuming fresh fruits, meats, vegetables, and grain carbohydrates.

Almond Milk

There was a time that the word "milk" was always equated with milk from a cow. Today, milk is a more generic term that can refer to milk derived from other sources, such as soy and almonds.

The good news is that the food industry is constantly evolving and changing, and responding to the demand for lower-calorie options. Today, I encourage people to explore the health benefits of almond milk. From a calorie perspective, almond milk can now be purchased that has only thirty calories per cup—more than a 60 percent calorie reduction over cow's skim milk. Almond milk is made from one of the most healthful nuts. It is also high in calcium, which all of us need for healthy teeth, bones, and overall bodily functions.

If you have lactose sensitivity or intolerance, then regular cow's milk, cheese, and ice cream may be causing you to have abdominal cramps, bloating, and diarrhea. Almond milk is lactose-free and will not lead to those problems.

Almond milk may be used in coffee and tea (served as both hot and cold beverages). Almond milk also combines with oatmeal to make for a great breakfast option on The OWL Diet. I like to combine almond milk with ice and fruit in a blender to create rich and filling smoothies.

My enthusiasm for the health benefits of almond milk means that it is now allowed on today's smarter OWL Diet plan. You will learn how to do a calorie exchange between almond milk and fruit.

Almond milk ranges in calorie count from a low of thirty calories per cup to a high of ninety calories per cup. Read the label with care to ensure that you are using the thirty-calorie-per-cup almond milk on the diet.

Alcohol

When I lost weight on this program I was drinking wine on a daily basis. I found that I could have one glass of wine per day and still succeed at losing weight. If I could drink a glass of wine every day and still lose weight, then I thought other people should be given the same opportunity.

Today, I have made the personal choice to no longer consume alcoholic beverages. At this stage in my life I have found that, for me, there are more negatives than positives to the use of alcohol. I recognize that many people continue to

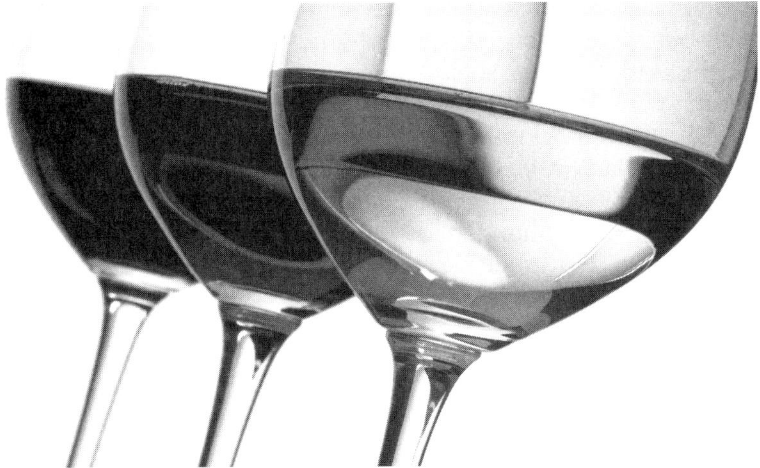

One four ounce glass of dry wine can be exchanged for the daily 100-calorie bread allowance.

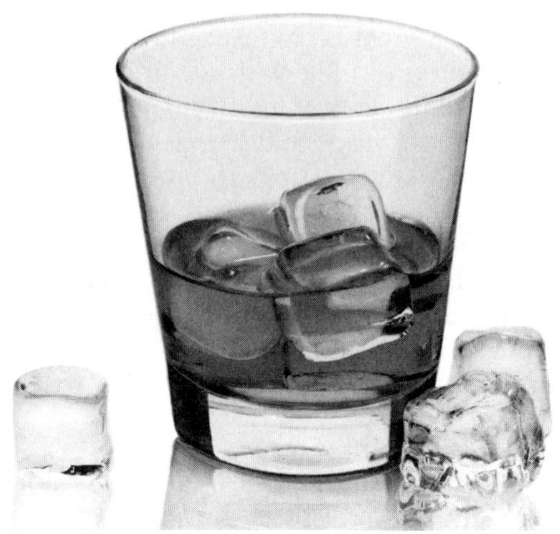

One and one-half ounces serving of liquor or spirits—such as whiskey, rye, vodka, tequila, gin, or rum—is approximately 100 calories.

drink alcohol in moderation with great success and satisfaction. In several clinical studies, moderate alcohol use has been demonstrated to have certain health benefits.

Alcohol also plays a social role in our society. Many people drink alcohol while socializing with friends and family. Alcohol is often consumed at sporting events and is often incorporated into business functions. In fact, the prevalent position that alcohol holds in our social life can make its avoidance during dieting very difficult!

I am not promoting or condoning the use of alcohol. But for a diet plan to be successful, it needs to appeal to the broad number of people who choose to drink alcohol. Therefore, an allowance for alcohol had to be a feature of The OWL Diet plan. With that in mind there are very specific rules to the accepted use of alcohol on my diet plan. The diet allows approximately 100 calories of alcohol per day. Because my "bread or grain" allowance per day also approximates 100 calories, it is an easy exchange to make. Most beers and spirits are made from grains, so this exchange also makes intuitive sense.

If you choose to have alcohol on The OWL Diet, please follow these simple rules:

- Alcohol is a "have it or lose it" allowance every day—you cannot bank them up and have several drinks on one day.
- Choose one serving of alcohol that is approximately 100 calories per day.
- On a day you choose to have an alcoholic beverage you will not be allowed to have a serving of "bread or grain"—this is an exchange between the two groups.
- You must choose your alcoholic drink from my approved list.

Choose one of the following approved drinks as a single serving:

- 4 ounces of dry wine—white or red
- 1½ ounces of liquor or spirits—such as whiskey, rye, vodka, gin, or rum
- A 12-ounce serving of a "light beer" (read the label to ensure it is no more than 100 calories per serving)

Proteins: Meats, Eggs, Tofu, and Beans

When I mention the word "meat" to patients most of them think of "beef." My definition of meat that is approved for use on The OWL Diet consists of a variety of lean meat choices including lean ground beef, lean beef steaks, white chicken, white turkey, white fish, shrimp, and scallops. You will also learn about lean "game" meat options (bison and venison), egg whites, and the use of tofu and beans as vegetarian options.

In the nutrition world there has been a long-standing tradition to calculate the calorie value of meat from a raw weighed portion. We continue that trend and ask you to weigh your meat raw, before cooking (exceptions are canned tuna packed in water, precooked shrimp, and canned crab meat packed in water).

Having you weigh your meat before cooking will also teach you to shop for uncooked meats and learn how to prepare them at home. Precooked meats are convenient, but less healthful for you. Meats that are cooked for you at the grocery

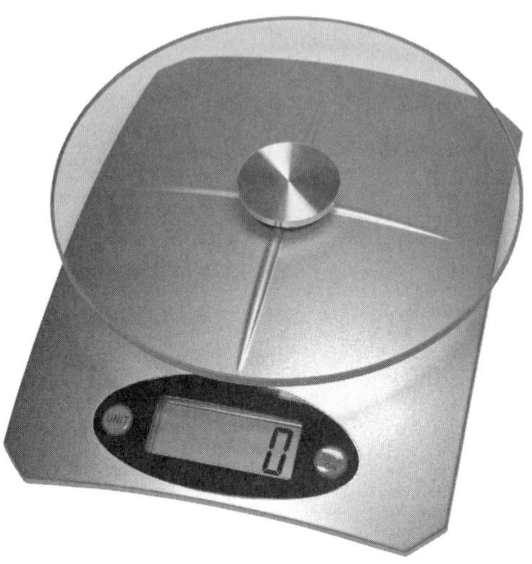

Obtain a reliable food scale to weigh your meat and protein prior to cooking.

store or in a food factory may have incorporated the use of oils, additives, and preservatives.

Weigh the meat on a food scale before you cook it. The older type of spring scale with a basket will work just fine, as will a digital scale. Some digital scales have a "tare" function that allows you deduct the weight of a container used to hold the food while it sits on the scale.

On The OWL Diet, meat is listed under the following categories:

- seven-ounce per day options
- five-ounce per day options
- egg whites
- vegetarian options

Seven-Ounce per Day Meat Choices

- Beef—ground beef (no less than 97 percent lean)
- Chicken—white meat only. Choose breast or tenderloin ("tenders"). Remove the skin and any visible fat before cooking. (When you cook chicken at home it then stores well for several days in the refrigerator, and may be rewarmed or eaten cold —such as diced and placed on a salad.)

- Turkey—white meat only. Remove the skin and any visible fat before cooking. (You may also purchase ground white turkey meat that will be labeled as more than 97 percent lean, but you must cook it yourself.)
- Shrimp—raw or precooked. (Precooked shrimp is pink in color and an excellent choice to make when your food prep time is limited.)
- White fish—any white fish, such as tilapia, orange roughy, perch, halibut, cod, catfish, northern pike, and others. (Precooked tuna packed in water will work, but is a bit higher in calories, so use it only twice per week.)
- White crabmeat— canned or fresh; precooked is fine.
- Bison and venison—raw (lean cuts only)
- Scallops—raw

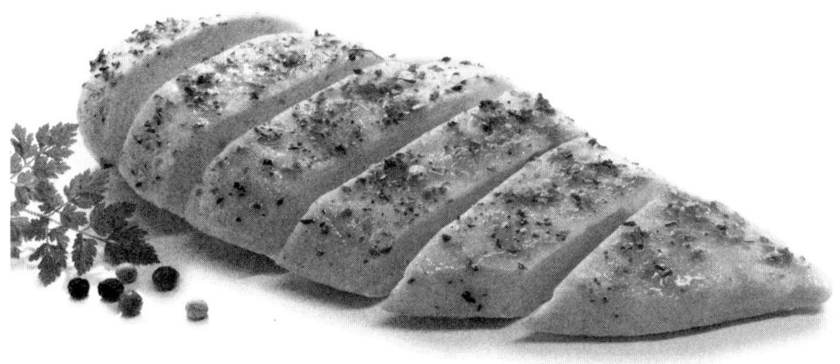

Seven ounces of chicken that has been weighed, seasoned, and then cooked, provides a lean source of protein to be divided into two meals.

Five-Ounce per Day Meat Choices

- Beef steak—raw cuts of only the leanest of steaks are allowed (free of all visible fat), such as filet mignon, strip, sirloin, or beef tenderloin
- Salmon—raw

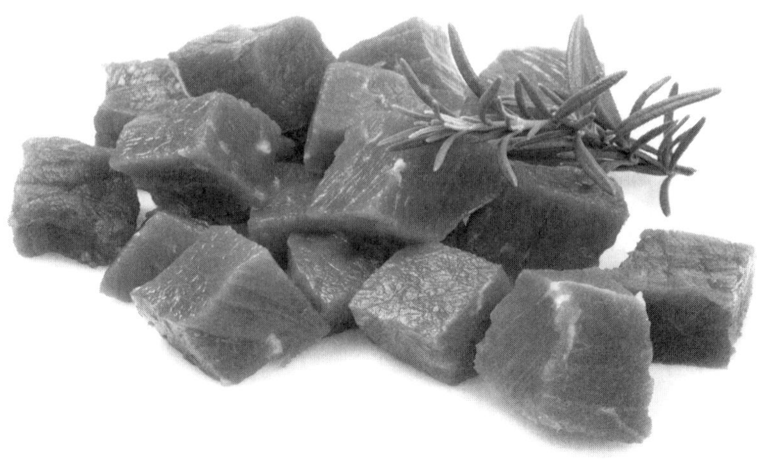

Here's what 5 ounces of uncooked, cubed lean beef looks like. Always weigh your meats on a food scale prior to cooking.

Egg White Substitute for "Meat"

Egg whites are low in calories and are frequently used as part of breakfast on The OWL Diet. The yolk is not allowed—it is high in both calories and cholesterol. A single-serving size of egg white that exchanges for 1 ounce of meat is:

- The whites of two medium-sized eggs
- ¼ cup of egg whites from a carton. (Read the calorie label to confirm that ¼ cup is no more than 30–40 calories.)

Vegetarian Substitute for "Meat"

A source of protein allowing 200 to 250 calories per day is needed for optimal fat burning. The vegetarian sources of protein that will work are:

- Beans—1 cup per day of uncooked navy, kidney, or white beans (Bake your own beans.)
- Tofu—7 ounces per day

Prepare Proteins Ahead

Once you have selected your protein options, I suggest that you precook enough protein to last you for several days. Remember to use your food scale for uncooked meat. Follow the proper five-ounce or seven-ounce limit, depending on your meat selection.

There are several cooking methods that work well:

- Cook on the stove in nonstick frying pans.
- Poach meat in a pot or pan of boiling water.
- Bake in the oven using a cookie sheet covered in foil.
- Use your indoor or outdoor grill.
- Some seafood can be "cooked" without heating, by using lemon or lime juice (ceviche).

The following meat may be purchased precooked:

- Tuna packed in water
- Shrimp that has been steamed in water prior to purchase
- Crab meat packed in water

Divide your portion of meat or protein equally into two meals. By dividing your meat into two meals, you will have better hunger control, better energy, and a better fat burn.

The consumption of protein is an important part of the fat-burning process. You may not omit this group of foods. You may mix your variety of meats eaten in a given day, for example by having 3.5 ounces of chicken at lunch, and 3.5 ounces of white fish for supper.

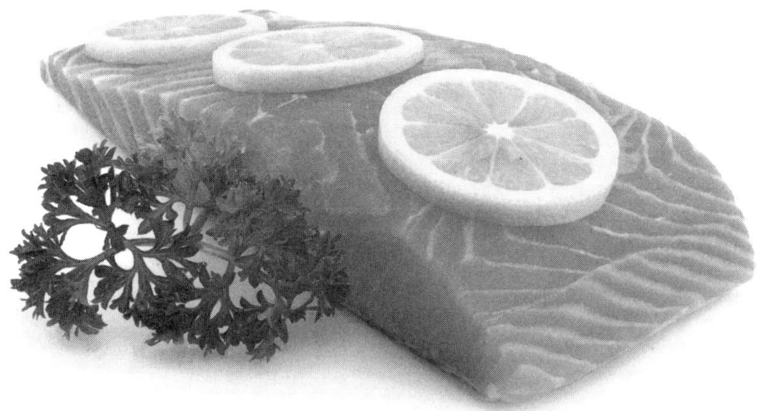

Salmon is allowed on The OWL Diet; however, count 5 ounces as your total daily protein allowance.

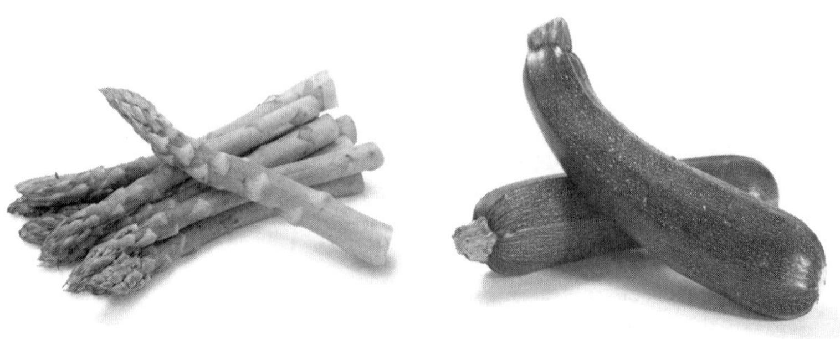

One cup of asparagus or zucchini, measured raw, are among your daily vegetable choices.

Proteins for Lunch and Supper

You will divide your protein choices into two meals per day. I call these two meals lunch and supper. What do you eat with your protein at these two meals? The answer is vegetables! Ideally, you will make two salads per day. A great plan is to add one cup of fresh vegetables on top of two cups of salad greens and eat that twice per day with your protein allowance. That will leave you with two more cups of fresh vegetables that can then be eaten raw as snacks or cooked for eating at lunch and supper.

Vegetables

The daily allowance of fresh vegetables is four cups per day (measured raw, before cooking). All vegetables are allowed except for corn and potatoes. Choose at least four different vegetables every day. (The calorie count of vegetables varies, so by eating a variety of vegetables the calorie count averages out nicely.) Some of your four-cup vegetable allowance will be used to make salads. This should leave some vegetables to enjoy raw as snacks, or cooked with your meals. Choose from:

- tomatoes
- radishes
- cucumbers
- broccoli
- peppers (of any color)
- onions
- zucchini
- cauliflower

- squash
- green beans
- cabbage
- mushrooms
- snow peas
- asparagus
- Brussels sprouts

Some vegetables are higher in calories than others, so the key is to limit each vegetable choice to no more than one cup per day of that particular vegetable. For example, no more than one cup of higher-calorie squash, carrots, peas, or onions per day. Try to have a salad twice per day, typically at lunch and supper with your meat or protein choices.

The "green leaf" salad options include iceberg (head) lettuce, romaine, baby leaf, spinach, arugula, and mixes of greens with fresh herbs. Your "green leaf" selection is limited to four cups per day (two cups twice per day). (Four cups of "green leaf" is very low in calories, helps your stomach to feel full, and works to keep your bowels regular—the reason that "green leaf" is not counted as part of your 800 calories per day.)

Select fresh vegetables to place atop the "green leaf" salad—such as tomatoes, cucumbers, radishes, bell peppers (any color), mushrooms, thin shavings of carrot, and peas. Choose Walden Farms brand of salad dressings to use on your salad. They are calorie-free, lactose-free, sugar-free, and gluten-free.

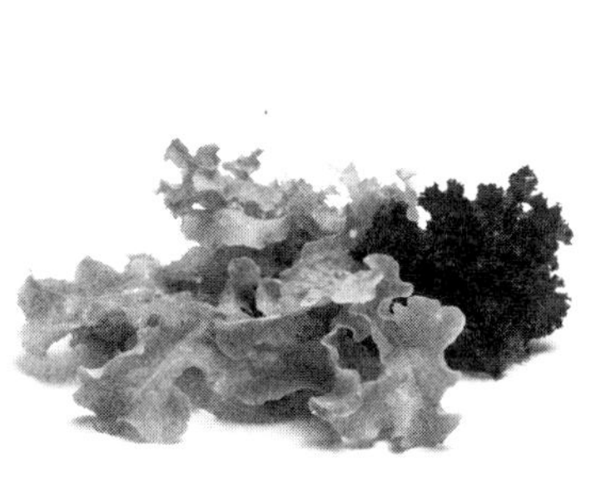

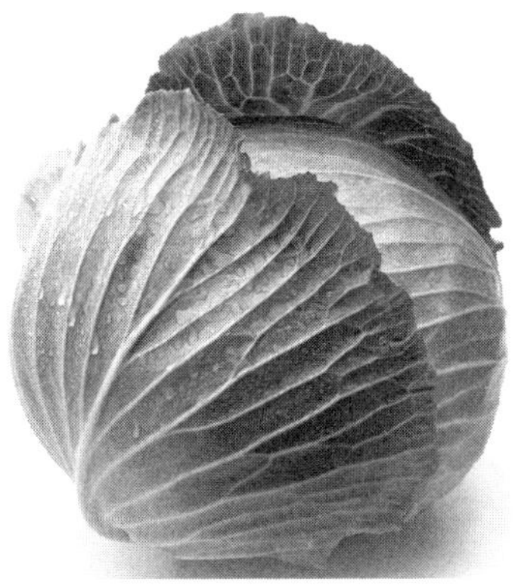

You may use two cups of leaf lettuce twice per day in addition to four cups of other approved raw vegetables.

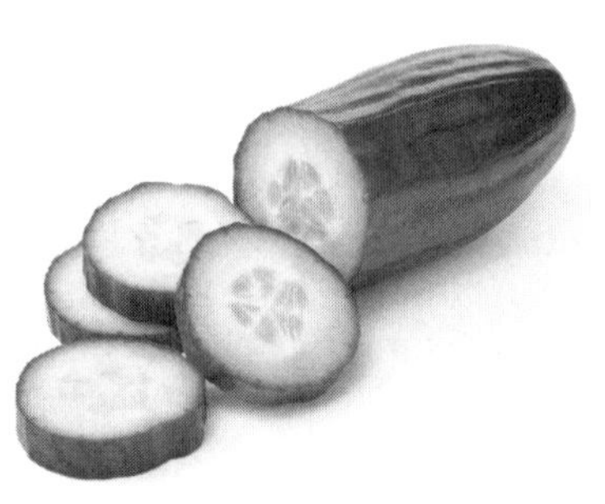
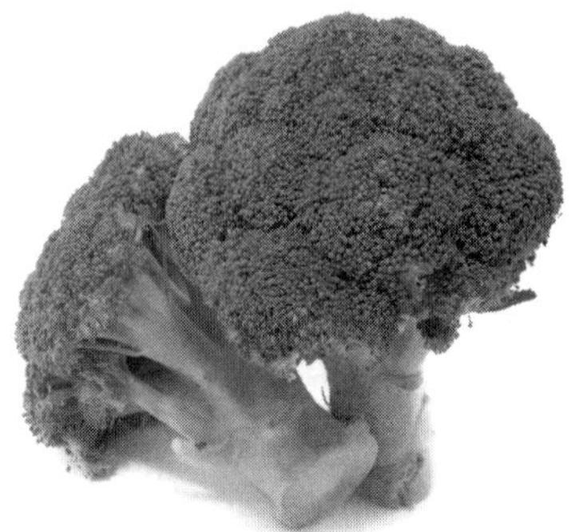

Eating the same vegetables can become boring—choose from a variety. Eat four cups of vegetables, measured before cooking, each day.

"Free" Vegetables

Celery is "free" food, and makes a fiber-rich snack food between meals. Dill pickles are "free" food and make a good snack between meals. Dill pickles are cucumbers preserved in white vinegar. When they are stored in glass containers at room temperature, dill pickles are rated calorie-free. If the pickles are "cold-packed" (kept in the refrigerator prior to opening) then they will usually be listed as "five calories per serving."

Caution: If you have high blood pressure (hypertension) or heart failure, then you must limit your salt intake. Pickles are high in salt and should be used with caution, or not at all. No one should consume more than two dill pickles per day.

Fruits

You are allowed three servings of fruit per day. Fruit makes for great snacks to be enjoyed mid-morning, afternoon, and in the evening before bed. Some participants use a full serving of fruit as part of their breakfast. You may use a variety of different OWL-approved fruits every day.

The following are single servings of fruit (all are measured raw, before cooking):

- 1 medium-sized apple, orange, nectarine, peach, or pear
- 2 small clementine oranges

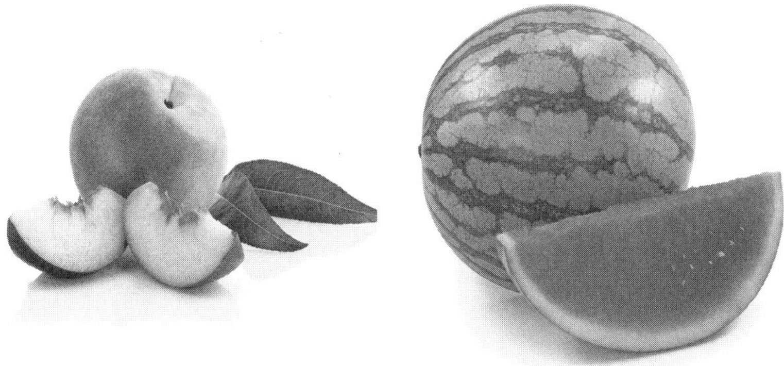

You have a wide variety of fresh fruits to choose for your daily servings.

- 1 cup of fresh blueberries, raspberries, blackberries, or sliced strawberries
- 1½ cups of diced melon such as honeydew, cantaloupe, or watermelon
- 1 whole grapefruit (Caution: grapefruit may interact with some prescribed medications; consult your health care provider before consuming grapefruit.)
- 2 small kiwis

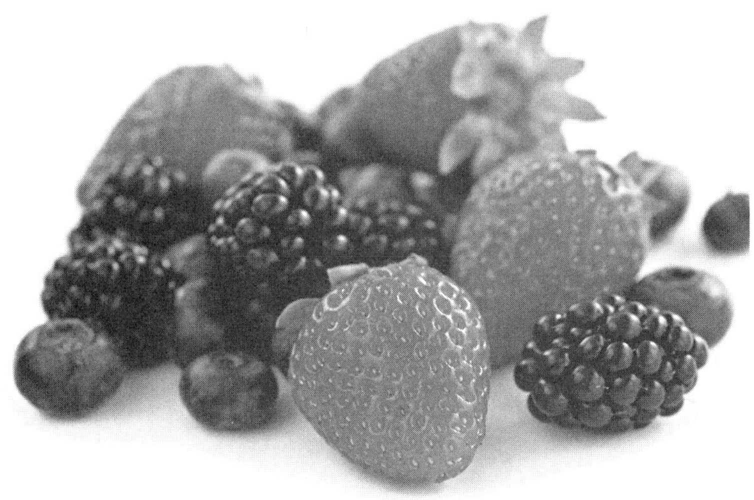

One cup of fresh berries makes up one of your fruit choices for the day.

Fruit Substitutions

If you wish, you can "trade" a fruit choice for almond milk or yogurt on The OWL Diet, but remember these are "exchanges" or substitutions for fruit choices. One serving of fruit may be exchanged with one of the following:

- a serving of yogurt that totals 80–90 calories
- almond milk that totals 80–90 calories. (Purchase almond milk that is labeled as 30 calories per cup and use up to 3 cups per day—by itself, perhaps combined with oatmeal, in a smoothie, or in coffee/tea.)

Grain and Bread Products

Many people are surprised to find that I allow one serving of a bread product on The OWL Diet. I believe that it is unrealistic to ask people to follow a diet that does not allow any grain or bread as part of their daily intake.

The daily "bread or grain" allowance is approximately 100 calories. The most popular choices are listed on the next page. There are other products you may find that also meet the 100-calorie limit but please read the calorie label with great care when making your selections. A single-day allowance of bread/grain includes:

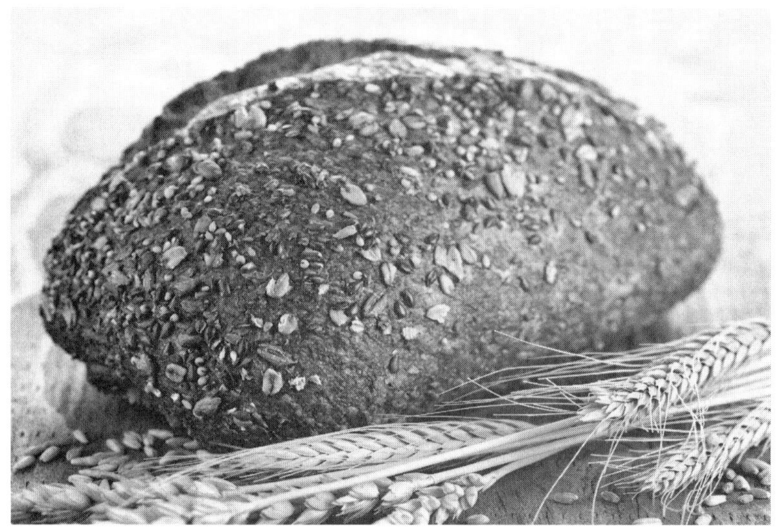

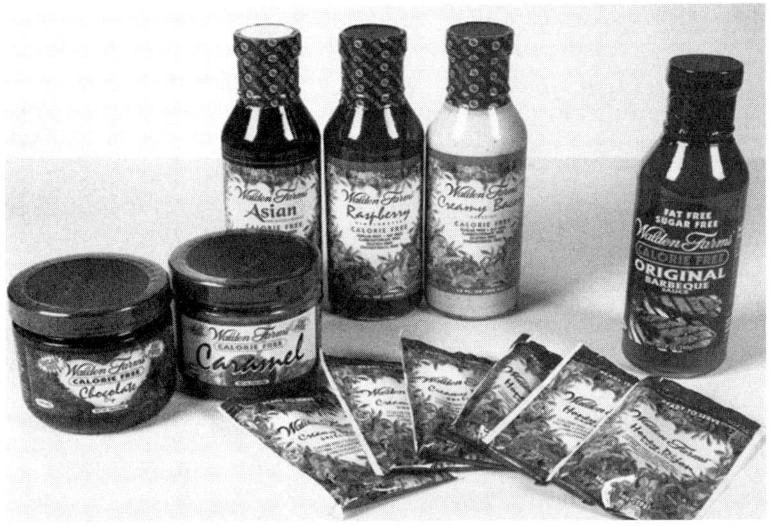

Explore the variety of products offered by the Walden Farms brand. Their products, which contain zero calories, include: salad dressings, dips, syrups, and fruit spreads.

- Melba toast—5 pieces of Melba toast (Avoid the rounds, which are too oily; choose the traditional shape which is rectangular.)
- Bagel Thins (Thomas' brand)
- Thin buns or sandwich thins (Oroweat or Earth Grains brand)
- Italian breadsticks—a great snack between meals, may be crumbled onto salads, or crushed and used to coat chicken or fish. (You are allowed four Alessi brand breadsticks—garlic, plain, or sesame flavored. For other brands of breadsticks, read the label to correctly select a 100-calorie portion.)
- Ak-Mak crackers— 1 sheet of 4 crackers is a 1-day allowance
- 100-calorie bag of microwaveable popcorn—94 percent fat-free
- 40- to 45-calorie thin-sliced bread (Pepperidge Farms, Sara Lee)—2 slices per day
- Wasa crackers—read the package and limit to a total of 100 calories per day

- Quaker oatmeal "one-minute oats"—measure ¼ cup before cooking. Add ½-cup almond milk (30 calories per cup), then microwave on high for 60–75 seconds. Add calorie-free cinnamon and sweetener (Splenda or others) for taste.

Note: A single serving of alcohol may be exchanged for one serving of bread daily.

Oils

The OWL Diet is low in oils, due to their high calorie count. Even in maintenance, it is important for you to limit your use of oils in cooking. Try the following for nonstick cooking and for a buttery flavor.

- Nonstick cooking sprays—multiple brands, including PAM. (A quick spray–1/3 of a full spray–is rated as zero calories.)
- Smart Balance spray or I Can't Believe It's Not Butter spray. These sprays are a soy by-product and are rated as zero calories per spray. (Limit yourself to ten sprays per day to be on the safe side.)

Dressings, Vinegars, and Condiments

Today, there are a number of low-calorie or no-calorie dressings and condiments you can purchase to help you maintain the right number of calories without feeling deprived of flavors.

Here are examples:

- Walden Farm's calorie-free products—salad dressings, BBQ sauce, caramel dip, chocolate dip.
- Bragg Liquid Aminos is a zero-calorie soy sauce, great for flavoring meat or stir-fried vegetables.
- Cider vinegar and rice wine vinegar are zero calories.
- Vinegars such as balsamic and wine vinegars are low calorie, and may be used in moderation. The same is true for Worcestershire sauce.
- "Southern-style" hot sauces (Tabasco, Cholula, and others) are calorie-free.
- Regular mustard is calorie-free (French's).

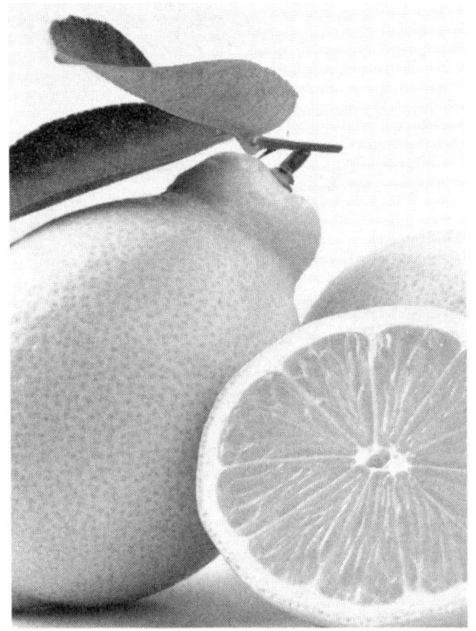
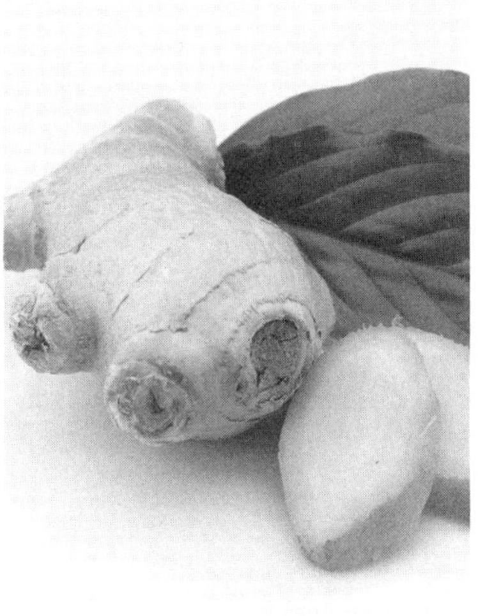

Enhancing food flavors makes eating more enjoyable. Brighten flavors with fresh lemon juice or grated ginger.

- Seasonings and spices, fresh or dried herbs, and curry are fine. Garlic is safe to use in moderation.
- Lemon and lime concentrates are considered calorie-free (RealLemon, RealLime). If you want to use a fresh lemon or lime, use no more than one per day (1 lemon or 1 lime is about 10 calories).
- Artificial sweeteners—Splenda, Sweet'NLow, Equal, Truvia, Stevia, and others are all acceptable to use.
- Consider using beef or chicken stocks in moderation. Check the calorie allowance and use no more than 10 calories per day in this category.
- Pickled peppers such as yellow banana and cherry peppers are low in calories and make for a great snack, or addition to lunch and supper. (Limit use if you are sensitive to salt.)
- Make your own salsa, without adding oil. There are now store brands of fresh salsa that are also low in calories and can be used in moderation (carefully read the calorie label). Count ½-cup of fresh salsa as 1 cup of the fresh vegetable allowance.

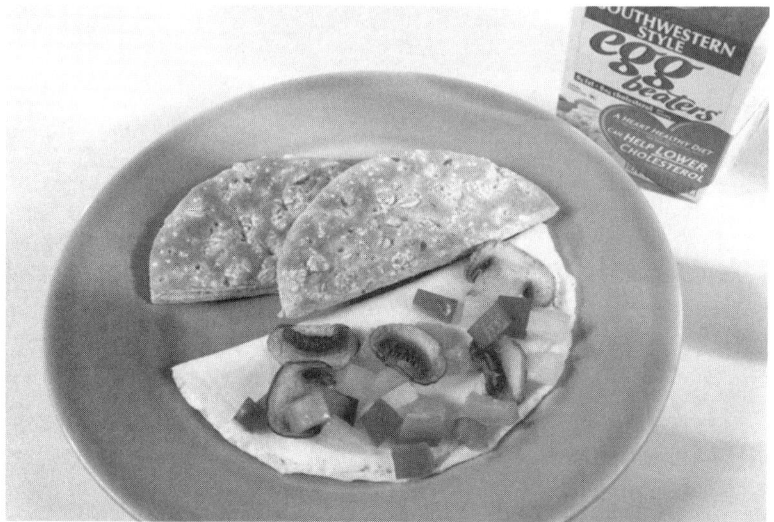

Omelets, made of egg whites or Egg Beaters, are a popular breakfast choice. Enhance flavor with mushrooms, onions, or peppers.

Breakfast Suggestions

On The OWL Diet, breakfast is mandatory as one of your three daily meals. Here are some popular options:

- Make a fruit smoothie—Combine fruit, ice cubes, and almond milk in a blender. Add artificial sweetener, nutmeg, and cinnamon as desired.
- Egg-white omelet—Dice fresh vegetables such as peppers, mushrooms, onions, and tomatoes then stir-fry in a nonstick pan. Combine with the whites of 2 medium-sized eggs or ¼-cup of Egg Beaters for a small omelet (1-ounce meat exchange). Top with salt, pepper, or hot sauce. May be combined with toasted Bagel Thin, sandwich thin, or thin-sliced bread.
- Use sugar-free jam in moderation (limit to a 10-calorie portion per day).
- Have a serving of fruit.
- Have a serving of 80-calorie yogurt (exchanges for 1 serving of fruit).
- Instant oatmeal—¼ cup of oatmeal with ½-cup of low-calorie almond milk equals 100 calories and is your "grain/bread" allowance for the day

9

"I'm Not Losing Weight"

The OWL Diet does not fail people, but people don't always succeed on The OWL Diet. Weight loss is not easy. Staying focused and committed to the plan is critical to succeeding on this low-calorie diet averaging 800 calories per day. There are several reasons why those on The OWL Diet do not succeed.

The Wrong Timing

Timing is important! Losing weight is not a race—it's a journey. You are reading this book because you feel a sense of urgency to start a weight-loss program. But resist the temptation to get started too quickly. First, learn the plan and then choose the right date for you to start The OWL Diet.

If you have travel plans in the immediate future, delay your start until after you return from your trip. Look at the next month. Do you have any birthdays, holidays, graduation parties, weddings, or other functions that you must attend over the next month? If so, you may want to get those events in the rear-view mirror before focusing on the diet.

Do you have any personal health issues that might impact your ability to follow the diet plan? Examples may include upcoming minor or major surgeries, or starting new prescription medications. Try to find a time that your personal health is relatively stable. If, on the other hand, your current health is unstable because of your obesity, then it's necessary to get going on OWL Diet success right now!

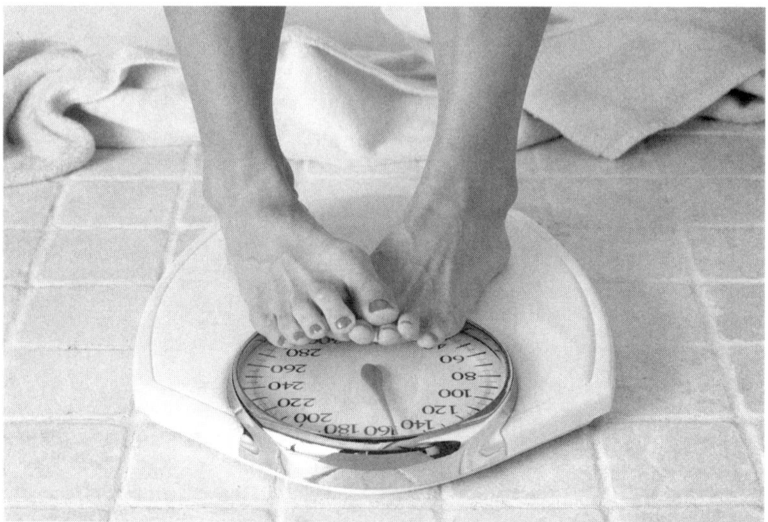

For many of us, keeping off excess weight is a life-long challenge. I recommend weighing yourself daily. Your weight can fluctuate, but if you gain back ten pounds, I suggest you take action and go back on The OWL Diet for a month.

During initial consultations, I do my best to get people to answer this question really honestly: "Is this a good time in your life to commit to losing weight?"

Personal situations that raise red flags include:

- A recent diagnosis of depression or anxiety
- The start of new psychotropic medications (for mood disorder)
- A recent life stressor such as starting a new job, a move, loss of a loved one, or new health problems
- Recent separation or divorce
- Having just quit smoking
- The need for frequent travel or restaurant dining

On the other hand, one can *always* argue that you could always find an excuse why it is never a good time to lose weight! People with medical problems that are aggravated by obesity may have been advised that they can no longer delay efforts to lose weight.

For some of us, weight loss is part of reinventing ourselves. Divorce or job loss may help speed the decision to commit to The OWL Diet. Weight loss is often associated with improved self-esteem and enhances existing relationships. Controlling obesity may improve your chances of finding employment or a partner in life.

In every culture, there are events throughout the year that are associated with increased food consumption. It is easy to overeat and gain weight during these times. Such events include birthdays, anniversaries, holidays, and vacations. These events create potential roadblocks during dieting, and raise the risk of "cheating" (taking in extra food or calories that are not part of The OWL Diet program).

I have been on every diet known to man. I have even had the lap band surgery to help with my overeating, but I was still having a problem with my addiction to sugar. Then, I found Dr. Abbott. Being a nurse, I had plenty of questions for him. This program taught me how to eat real food, no shakes or bars. I lost forty-seven pounds in about two months!
Heidi, 37

Uncontrolled feelings of hunger may also be a sign that you are not ready to commit to The OWL Diet. You may have *thought* you were ready, and you certainly want to succeed, but your life situation may make it especially difficult to adjust to the sacrifices that go with consuming considerably fewer calories. It is important to frankly assess your current life situation to determine if this is the right time for you to commit to The OWL Diet. Let's face it, The OWL Diet requires not only commitment but sacrifice.

If your first effort to follow The OWL Diet did not go as well as expected, then set a new date to restart, focusing your activities, thoughts, and energy around adherence to the plan.

"I'm Still Hungry"

Despite the use of prescription medications to suppress their appetite, some participants still battle hunger cravings. As a survival mechanism, hunger that indicates a genuine need to eat for survival is a good thing. The OWL Diet allows you to

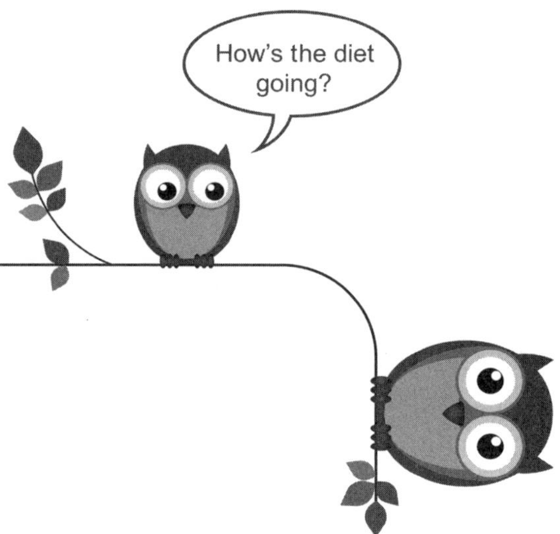

eat three meals per day, with snacks, and this will help manage genuine hunger.

But why do some dieters still feel hungry or the desire to eat all of the time? Realize that food cravings and the overwhelming desire to eat all starts in your brain. The brain is a sensory receptor for everything that is happening around us at all times. People who lead very active social lives tend to face a greater level of temptation to eat the wrong foods and beverages and eat too much. Having friends and supporters in your life is part of the key to lifelong happiness and better health. But regular social interaction with friends and family often tends to be equated with sharing food and beverages. When you socialize with other people, chances are very good that many of those gatherings will include dining in restaurants.

OWL dieters do not have to give up contact with other people, but they do need to find a balance between dieting success and staying connected with friends and family.

There are also many environmental triggers that create food temptations—ubiquitous fast food availability, TV advertisements, and attendance at live sporting events, to mention just a few. As our eyes send images to our brain, positive memories of eating certain foods can trigger an emotional desire to eat, even when we are not hungry.

Unexpected emotional issues may also be at work. Despite our best efforts during consultation to select the best time for a patient to start The OWL Diet, external stresses may develop such as family problems or changes at work. If this is the case, I suggest whether it might be in the best interests of the patient to take a pause in the program and start the diet again at a later date.

In some patients with hunger cravings, the addition of another prescribed appetite suppressant may be appropriate. Despite the benefits that may come from these medications, there may still be days of increased hunger. Hunger may occur on days three or four of the diet, or even several weeks later. Everyone is different. Part of your commitment to succeed has to be your willingness to work through the hunger.

When you experience hunger cravings, try the following:

- Distract your attention by changing activities.
- Drink a diet beverage or more water.
- Go for a walk.
- Call a friend for support.
- Eat a breadstick or have one of your allowed servings of fruit.
- Snack on a dill pickle or celery.

When you have your next weekly check-in visit and see an additional weight loss of three to four pounds, you will be glad that you stuck with the program!

Coping with Urges to Eat

Resisting the urge to eat draws on your motivation and requires you to manage your thoughts, feelings, and food behavior. You will not always be successful in controlling your urges, and that simply means you are not perfect. Although to err is human, too much cheating on the diet will result in the obvious consequence—the failure to lose any weight.

Many of us become overweight because we eat out of habit, not necessity. Our habit becomes a reflex action. We must enter into an internal dialogue about our urges to eat. The best way to do this is to think about the positive and negative consequences of eating the wrong foods, for example, the urge to eat cake and ice cream at a birthday party.

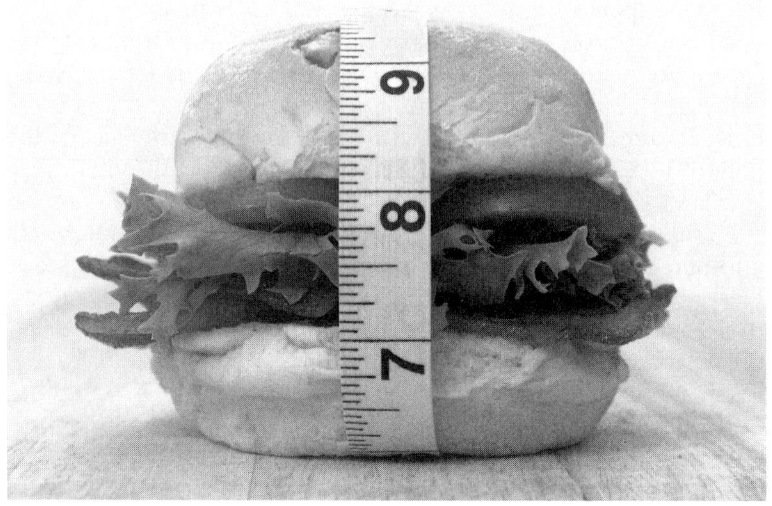

A sandwich containing bacon is certain to have negative consequences on the diet.

Positive consequences: I will enjoy the treat. I love the taste of cake and ice cream. I will be celebrating with other people and sharing in the event.

Negative consequences: I will not lose weight on the diet today, and I might even gain some weight. I might want to go back for a second serving. If I cheat now, will my urge to eat the wrong foods be even stronger tomorrow? If I continue to cheat, I won't lose any weight this week and I will feel disappointment in myself.

Engaging in this internal dialogue, weighing the pros and cons of the urge, will help you determine what your choice will be. The choice to eat or not eat the cake and ice cream is your own. By following this way of thinking, you are taking control over your urges.

Avoid High-Risk Situations

I suggest that you avoid eating in restaurants altogether during active dieting. It is very challenging to choose OWL Diet–approved foods from a restaurant menu.

When you are scheduled to meet with family and friends, try to avoid meeting around an eating activity. Consider other options, such as having people over to your home and offering healthful food choices. Find activities that you enjoy that do not revolve around food and alcohol.

Too Much Exercise

Despite my advice to the contrary, some OWL Diet participants engage in highly active forms of exercise. They may be running, riding a bicycle for an hour every day, walking more than two miles per day, or body-building with heavy weights. Others may be going to exercise classes or fitness training camps that push them to the upper limits of their abilities. Although it may seem intuitive to participants that increasing exercise, while following a calorie-restricted diet, will lead to even faster weight loss, the opposite typically occurs.

Most doctors have only criticized me rather than motivate me, but Dr. Abbott and his staff are so warm and caring. I have not once been criticized, not even on a bad weigh-in. I have experienced amazing results in a short amount of time—I lost 8 pounds in the first 4 days!
Sherrie, 34

Why is that? In my experience, excessive levels of physical activity negates all of the positive effects of hunger control that The OWL Diet program provides. Exercise that results in a markedly increased heart rate, increased respiration, or heavy sweating inevitably drives hunger. Hunger arising from exercise is hard to ignore and usually results in an increased intake of food, beyond that allowed with my program.

OWL dieters who exercise too much will typically state at their weekly visits that they are very hungry and had to eat more food (calories). I believe them when they tell me they are hungry! I would be, too, if I worked out as hard as they do. When they weigh in, they are disappointed to find that they did not lose weight or lost only one to two pounds over the last week. They are unintentionally sabotaging their own program.

The solution is simple. They need to slow down to the level of activity that is approved on The OWL Diet. The correct mild to moderate level of physical activity will maintain fitness and prevent muscle wasting. If they listen to my advice and get back to following the diet plan, they are then rewarded the following week with an acceptable weight loss.

If, on the other hand, they continue to insist on exercising more than is recommended, they will finish the month feeling miserable, complaining that they were hungry all month long, and be disappointed with a less-than-optimal amount of weight loss.

Cheating

"Cheaters" are those dieters who do not follow The OWL Diet protocol, eating extra calories that are not permitted. The result is no loss of weight or weight loss that is less than optimal.

There may be several reasons for this behavior:

- They chose the wrong time to start the diet.
- They may battle chronic low self-esteem and lack the confidence to succeed.
- They experience excessive emotional stress that triggers "comfort eating."
- They don't get enough sleep and the deprivation causes poor hunger control and a slower metabolism.
- They are repeating a self-destructive behavior pattern.
- Their level of commitment is not there.
- They lack the support of their spouse, friends, family, and coworkers.
- Depression or other emotional problems require treatment before they can succeed.
- They have an underactive thyroid condition that requires treatment.

Some cheaters are honest about consuming extra calories and admit this fact at their weekly visit. This group has the ability to let go of the previous week's failure, understand why they cheated, and work to recommit and follow The OWL Diet program as laid out for them. We all bend the rules sometimes and dieting is no exception. There should be no guilt or shame in having a bad week, as long as one strives to do better. These dieters earn my respect for being honest, and deserve as much support, encouragement, and coaching as they need.

Other cheaters try to hide the fact that they consumed extra calories. This group of people will not do well, as they fail to assume responsibility for their choices. They will typi-

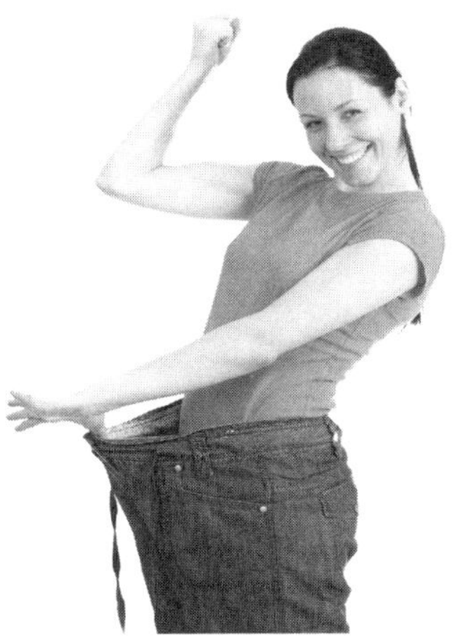

The OWL Diet does not fail people, but people can fail on the diet. Be consistent and you will be rewarded!

cally transfer the blame to The OWL Diet plan in general, and the health care providers associated with the diet program. Ultimately, the dishonest cheater will choose to stop The OWL Diet program and I usually never hear from them again. For the diet cheaters who do not take responsibility for their choices, this will be "just another diet that did not work." They are only cheating themselves of the opportunity to finally achieve permanent weight loss.

Whatever the cause or excuse for cheating, the reality is that no one forces us to eat. It is our own brain and our hand-to-mouth behavior that leads to diet cheating. It is our conscious decision to eat.

If you follow The OWL Diet faithfully, you will lose weight. This is simple arithmetic. When your body takes in 800 or even 1,000 calories in a day, it is looking for an additional source of energy to function and maintain life. Your body will use fat deposits to generate that additional energy and you will lose weight.

The only exception to this reality would be a patient with severe, undiagnosed hypothyroidism (underactive thyroid). If hypothyroidism is suspected, I would advise the patient to have his or her thyroid function checked, which is easily done with blood testing. A borderline thyroid result would not explain the inability to lose weight on The OWL Diet.

On a positive note, most people do commit to the OWL program, and reap the rewards of rapid and safe weight loss. The result is self-empowering. Nearly all the people we see are committed to the diet and are very happy with the results. This is a very positive program, with positive outcomes.

"Tweaking" the Diet

"Tweakers" are what I call people who add certain foods to The OWL Diet, even though the foods are not recommended or approved. At the initial consultation, when the diet is reviewed in detail, almost everyone asks to have certain foods added to the approved list. This negotiation is met with one or more of my standard responses:

- Don't set yourself up for failure before you even begin.
- Don't try to reinvent the wheel—the program works as it is set up so don't make changes to it.
- Put on blinders. Stay focused and stay committed.

"Tweaking" is what I call the behavior of adding unapproved foods to their diet with the hope of still losing weight at the typical rate seen on The OWL Diet. This behavior usually leads to disappointment at the scale.

Sometimes "cheating" is cloaked as "tweaking." Some people know they are cheating and that the extra calories will sabotage their weight loss, but they cloak the message to themselves and to others by saying they thought it would work, that the additional food would be fine, even though they know in their hearts it is not an approved food.

I want you to succeed. The OWL Diet today is smarter than ever, offering an expanded list of food options. Resist the temptation to tweak the diet.

Lack of a Support System

Despite their good intentions, your spouse, family, friends, and coworkers may be less supportive than you would like, or, worse, they may even attempt to sabotage your efforts at weight loss. The reasons for this behavior among friends and relatives are complex. Those who are sabotaging you might not even be aware of what they are doing. Below are a few possible interpersonal dynamics that you may face:

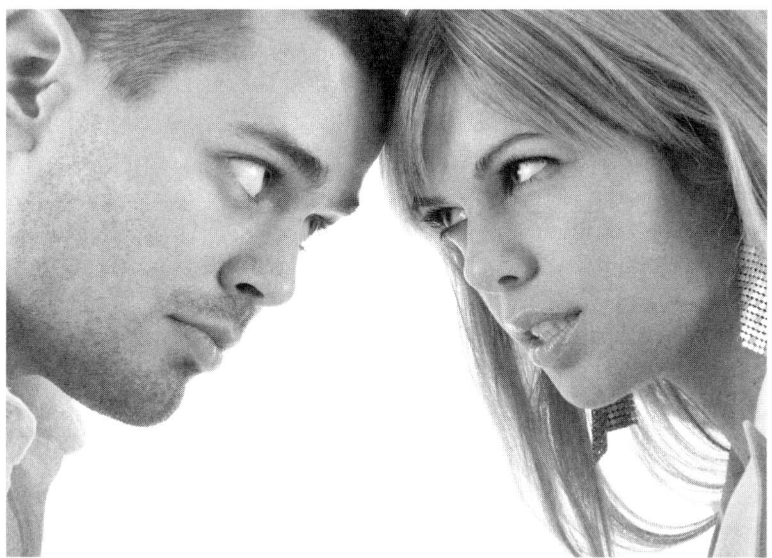

Be aware of how personal conflicts may affect your success on the diet.

Spouses

- They are more attracted to you as an overweight person.
- They feel threatened that you might leave them if you lose weight.
- They use the self-esteem that often accompanies being overweight to their advantage.
- If you lose weight, then they may have to lose weight also
- They like to eat out a lot.
- Dieting means not getting together with friends.
- They don't support you spending money on "another weight loss program."
- If you lose weight, you'll need more clothes, and that would mean spending more money.

Family and Friends

Many of the spouse sabotage strategies also apply here, but also:

- Worry this is a sign of an eating disorder (especially common in mothers).
- They are competitive about who looks best.
- They deny that you are actually overweight.
- They engage in control and power struggles with you—if you lose weight, you will prove that you are stronger.
- They complain that your dieting will ruin gatherings, especially during holidays.

Coworkers

Although many of the above sabotage strategies also apply to coworkers, the workplace may be one of the most potentially challenging environments, where some people act in hurtful ways due to:

- Competitiveness for better-paying jobs
- Competitiveness for attention of coworkers or senior staff

The workplace is also an area where you cannot control the food that is brought in by coworkers. It may be harder to

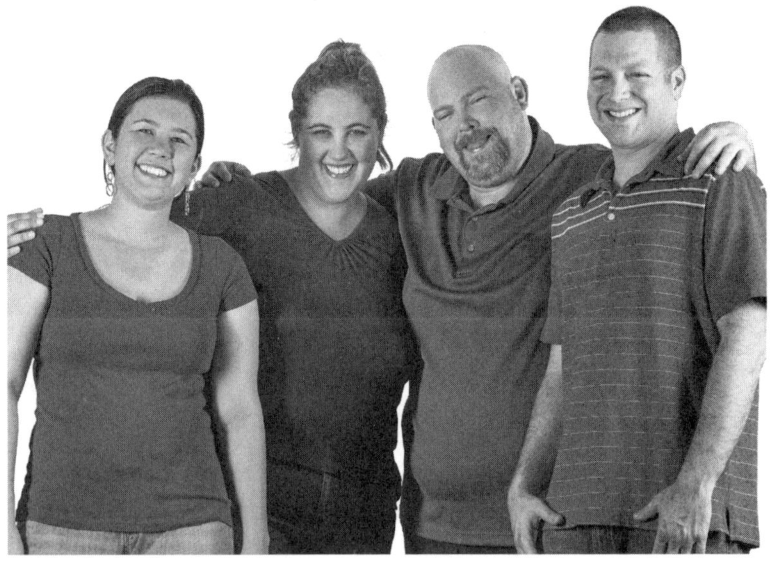

Who will be supportive, and who will be standing in the way of your weight loss success?

say "no" to a treat when you are at work and everyone else is enjoying a special snack or meal. If a coworker has brought in a home-baked item (perhaps your favorite treat), you may feel pressure to eat that food for fear of hurting your coworkers feelings.

Special events at work often include food treats, such as a going-away party for a staff member or seasonal holiday parties. Companies often use food to reward their employees for a job well done. As a society, we tend to shower food on one another as a way to celebrate or try to make the other person feel better.

The "Stealth Diet"

Due to concerns about how the people around you will react, some OWL Diet participants start out by keeping friends, family, coworkers, and even spouses in the dark about what they are doing. Reasons for concealing your diet plan also include your own fear of failure and perceived lack of support.

I do not recommend "stealth dieting" and keeping the fact that you are on The OWL Diet program a secret from everyone. You need to recruit all the support you can get to help you succeed. It is also important for you to identify where there may

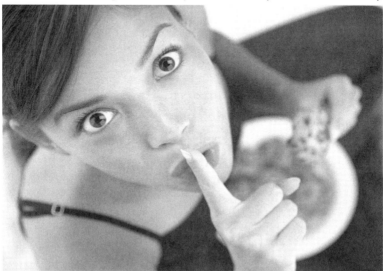

It is hard to keep your OWL Dieting a secret.

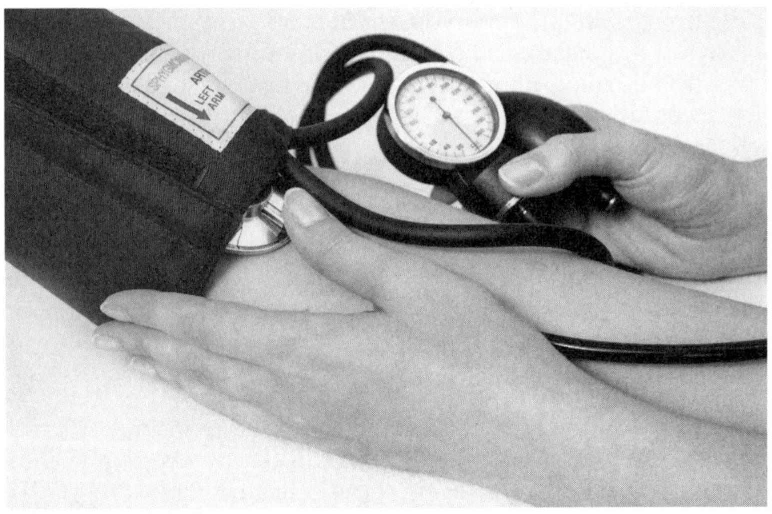

During your weekly support visits, we will monitor your blood pressure.

be lack of support. If you believe someone may try to sabotage your success, you need to plan for that possibility and how you will cope with it.

Being open with others about your weight-loss program also creates an increased accountability on your part. Don't take the approach, "I will try it for a few weeks to see how it goes." That attitude implies lack of commitment.

It is very hard to conceal The OWL Diet from your spouse, family, friends, and co-workers. The first clue will be the dramatic change in your eating habits. Concealing the use of prescription medications is equally challenging.

I recommend that you have a frank talk with the people in your life who need to know you are on The OWL Diet and ask them for their support. If you are reading this book, chances are you have already tried other diet plans that did not work for you. Previous lack of success leads to disappointment on your part, but may also create frustration in the people who love us the most.

Talk to the most important people in your life and explain why The OWL Diet is different from other diet plans. Explain to them that:

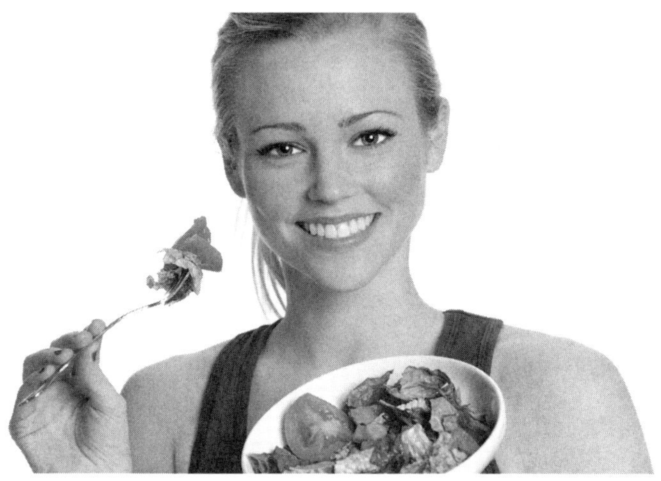

Our OWL Diet trained staff will help you shop, cook, and eat better.

- You will be getting the support of an office with health care workers.
- Your weight and blood pressure will be monitored weekly.
- You will have the option of using prescription medications.
- You will be learning to shop better, cook smarter, and limit meal portions—skills that will lead to permanent weight loss.
- You will be encouraged to engage in mild to moderate physical activity.

On a positive note, when your spouse, relatives, friends, and coworkers see how quickly you are losing weight, there is an excellent chance that they will be excited and pleased for you. They may even start The OWL Diet themselves, and join you on the journey to taking control over their own weight problems.

Let me add a final word on "buddies." A buddy can be an excellent partner to help you get through the bumps in the road that inevitably come along when you are changing life patterns. I do not recommend that you become an evangelist for

The OWL Diet. That tends to turn people off and turns up the volume of the complaints, cautions, and resistance. However, sometimes we choose friends who are of a similar weight, so if your social network or family has several overweight members, you might try asking one or two of them if they would like to join you on The OWL Diet. There is strength in numbers!

Part IV

OWL Wellness

10

Medical Conditions and The OWL Diet

Many of us have experienced serious medical conditions related to being overweight, such as diabetes, heart disease, and high blood pressure. It is not surprising that people with one or more of these serious medical conditions desire to undertake The OWL Diet. I can happily report that, for most of them, the results are positive and not only have they lost weight, they have improved their overall health.

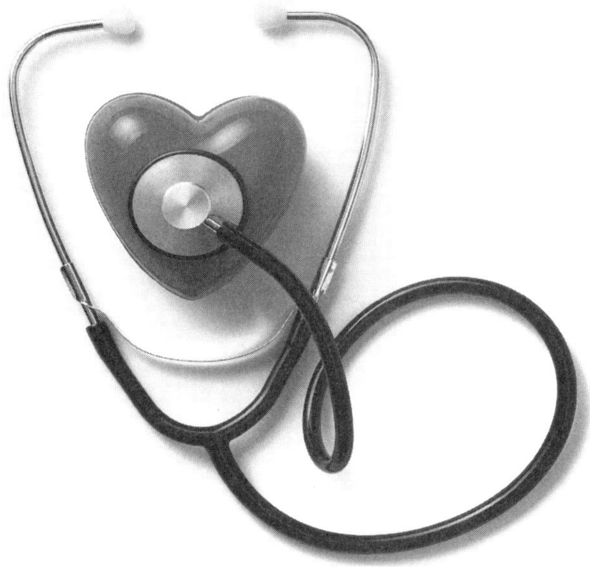

The OWL Diet is all about getting healthier.

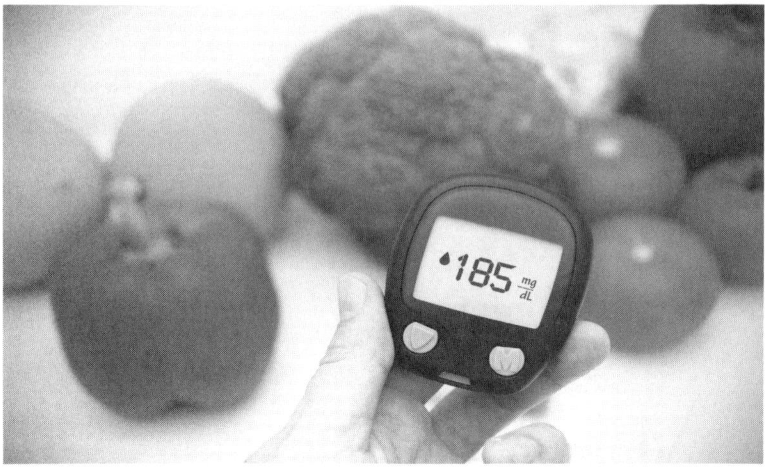

Diabetic patients are encouraged to monitor their blood sugars regularly while dieting.

In this chapter I will be making statements on a variety of medical conditions. These statements are my beliefs based upon my interpretation of current medical research combined with my clinical observations derived from thirty years of caring for patients. Medicine is an art as well as a science. This chapter reflects my professional opinions regarding the positive effects that weight loss can have on a variety of medical conditions. Always consult with a physician before undertaking any low-calorie diet and the use of prescription medications.

Diabetes Mellitus

Type 2 diabetes mellitus occurs in many overweight people. A problem called "insulin resistance" is typically present, whereby the body is producing insulin but defects occur at the cellular level that interfere with the functions that insulin normally performs. Often, the body is producing very high levels of insulin but it does not recognize insulin the way it should.

When an overweight person with type 2 diabetes loses weight, blood sugar control will typically improve, insulin resistance will decrease, and the need for diabetes medication will lessen. Any change in dose of diabetic medication needs to be made by your health care provider.

In some cases, by achieving a normal body weight, patients with type 2 diabetes may be able to stop diabetes medication altogether. They might even be told that they no longer have diabetes!

In some type 2 diabetics, the pancreas gland that produces insulin may eventually "burn out." If this happens, some of the oral diabetes medications will no longer be effective and patients will need to start insulin. The use of insulin helps the body process "sugars," which may in turn trigger an undesirable weight gain.

Omaha Med Spa has helped me lose weight and has helped me to learn the essentials to living a balanced and healthy life. Dr. Abbott and his team helped me lose more than 100 pounds, and I have maintained the weight loss now for over 10 months.

Terry, 36

Diabetics who are on insulin may participate in The OWL Diet. Once again, partnership with your health care provider is needed to carefully monitor medication requirements and interpret home-tested blood glucose results.

Type 1 diabetes mellitus is entirely different from type 2 diabetes. In type 1 diabetes the pancreas fails to produce enough insulin at the very onset of the disease. The result is low to absent levels of naturally produced insulin, and blood sugars that can rise to very dangerous levels. People diagnosed with type 1 diabetes will be placed on insulin for the rest of their lives.

At the time of diagnosis, most people with type 1 diabetes are not overweight, and may in fact have lost weight leading up to their diagnosis. With the institution of prescribed insulin in people with type 1 diabetes, any weight that was lost is typically recovered, and sometimes additional undesirable weight is gained.

With a healthful diet and regular activity, most type 1 diabetics are able to keep their weight at an ideal body mass index (BMI). However, some type 1 diabetics do become overweight and this can interfere with blood sugar control.

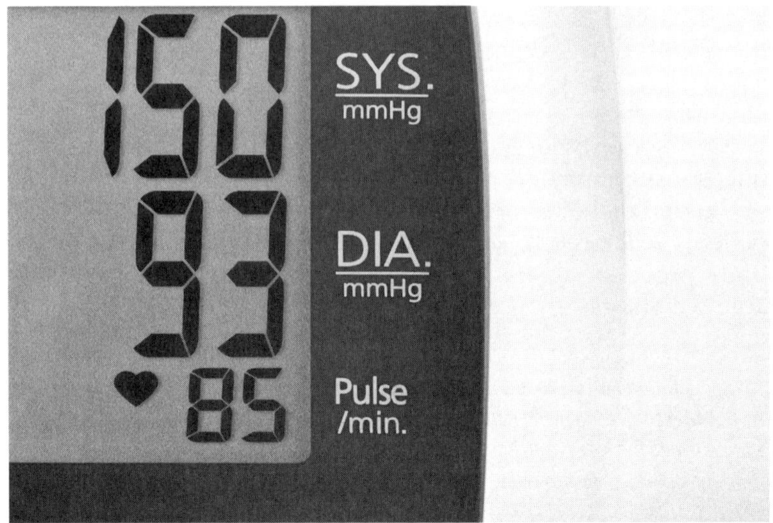

Patients with hypertension need to monitor their blood pressure as the need for medication may go down as they lose weight.

Patients with diabetes, and the people who live with them, need to know how to recognize the symptoms of low blood sugar (hypoglycemia) and have a clear plan on how to manage blood sugars that are too low.

Type 1 diabetics can participate in The OWL Diet, but only after careful consultation with the treating physician, regular home blood sugar testing, and regular visits with their health care provider. True type 1 diabetics will always require insulin, even after achieving an ideal body weight with the help of The OWL Diet plan.

Both type 1 and type 2 diabetics have been taught to follow a "diabetic diet," which is typically a balanced diet that is low in carbs and fats and promotes the consumption of lean meats. The OWL Diet has good news for diabetics: I promote all of those same food choices while dieting and in maintenance.

Hypertension

Elevated blood pressure (BP) is called hypertension. Obesity is a major risk factor for developing hypertension. Weight loss can have a profoundly beneficial effect on improving blood pressure. Frequent monitoring of blood pressure is necessary when you follow The OWL Diet. Losing weight, combined with eating more healthful foods, should improve your BP, and your need for BP-lowering medication may change. Any adjustment in the dose of your medication needs to be made by your health care provider.

In my experience, BP can improve quickly and dramatically in some hypertensive individuals as they lose weight. If you start developing symptoms of dizziness, light-headedness, or fatigue, then it may be a clue that your blood pressure is too low. You may find it helpful to purchase a device that allows you to check your blood pressure at home. If your BP drops too low, your health care provider may advise you to cut back on your medication.

The OWL Diet has helped me make a lot of changes in my life.
I lost a total of eighty-five pounds. I am eating better and so is my family.
Every week I have lost weight, and I am keeping it off.
Debbie, 59

Always remain well hydrated on The OWL Diet. Dehydration can also lead to the same symptoms as low blood pressure.

Obesity is only one of several risk factors for developing hypertension. Other factors include a positive family history of increased BP, smoking, lack of physical activity, and excessive sodium chloride (salt) intake. Limit your salt intake on The OWL Diet and consider using salt substitutes. Once you achieve your weight-loss goal, a regular exercise routine is also important for BP control.

Some people may have an ideal body weight but still have a diagnosis of hypertension, with the need for BP-lowering medications.

Hyperlipidemia

Hyperlipidemia means an increased level of fats or lipids in your bloodstream. There are many types and subtypes of lipids, but the main two for you to be familiar with are *cholesterol* and *triglycerides*. Different forms of hyperlipidemia have been linked to an increased risk of heart disease, stroke, poor limb circulation, pancreatitis, and dementia. Treating lipid dis-

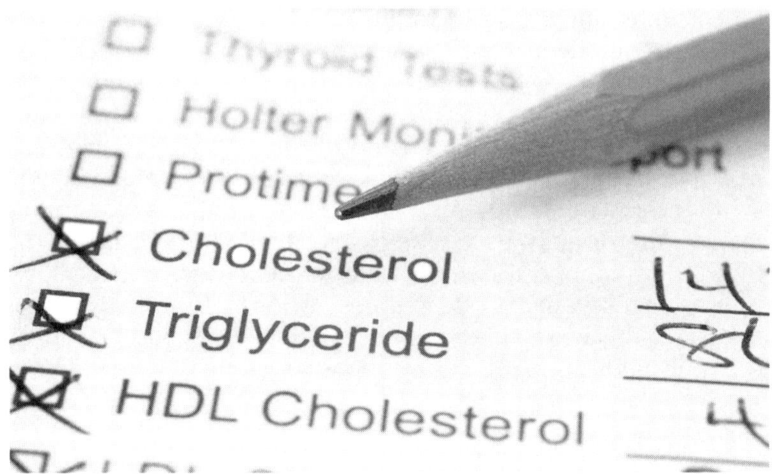

Cholesterol and triglyceride numbers will improve with weight loss.

orders may reduce the risk of these diseases, and many medications have been developed with that goal in mind. Elevated cholesterol is frequently caused by genetics. A family history of high cholesterol may genetically program you to overproduce cholesterol.

The effect of weight loss on lowering cholesterol is typically favorable, but the overall reduction may be less than ideal. People with a normal BMI and who eat a low-fat diet may still have elevated cholesterol, and may need to be on medication.

The OWL Diet is low in fat and oil. Continuation of a low-fat diet for life will help maintain your cholesterol at normal levels.

The other lipid of concern is triglycerides. Elevated triglyceride levels are closely aligned with obesity, but this condition also has a genetic basis. As your weight goes up, so do your triglycerides. Weight loss can play a very significant role in lowering triglycerides.

During The OWL Diet program, I typically recommend that you continue any prescribed lipid-lowering medications (such as "statins," "fibrates," niacin, or fish oil). If you have an established diagnosis of coronary artery disease, heart disease, peripheral arterial disease, or cerebrovascular disease (such as TIAs or strokes), then your doctor may not want you to stop your prescribed therapies.

Coronary Heart Disease

Coronary heart disease (CHD) occurs when there are blockages in the arteries that supply oxygen to the heart. Other names for CHD include coronary artery disease and arteriosclerosis. CHD may lead to angina pectoris, heart attack (acute coronary syndrome), and congestive heart failure.

If you have coronary heart disease, your doctor must determine that your heart health is stable before you are allowed to start The OWL Diet. The ketoacidosis (a drop in potassium that can affect your heart and muscles) that occurs with rapid weight loss of three or four pounds per week needs to be taken into consideration.

Your health care provider may determine that it is safer for you to follow a diet plan other than The OWL Diet. An alternate plan that leads to a more gradual loss of weight of one or two pounds per week may be more appropriate. Losing weight is not a race. The result is the same whether you take a slower or faster path to get there.

Thyroid Disease

The thyroid gland produces hormones that control the metabolic rate—the rate at which our body burns calories. If the thyroid gland is underactive, then not enough thyroid

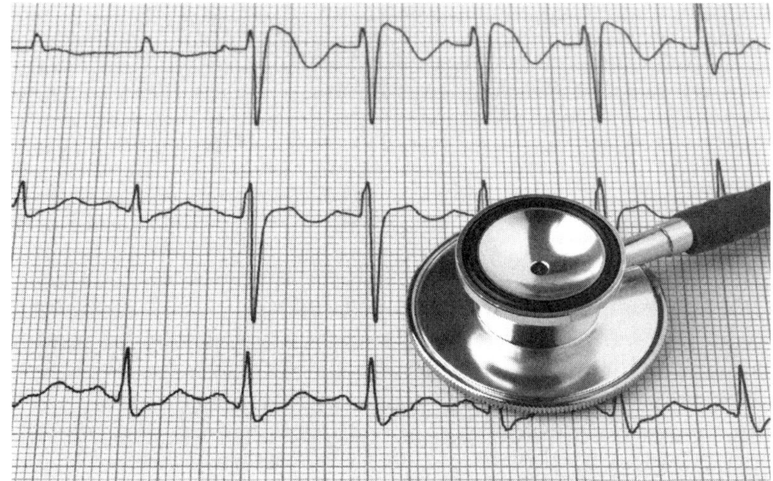

If you have heart disease, ask your doctor if the OWL Diet is right for you.

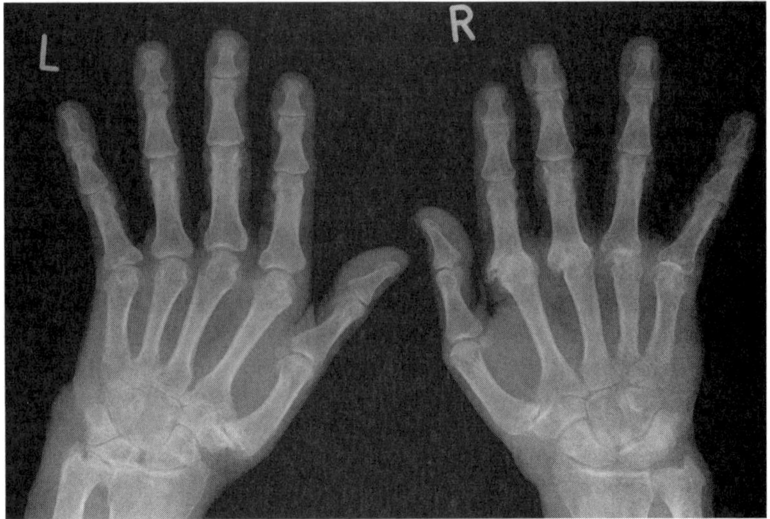

Arthritis in joints responds well to weight loss.

hormone is being produced and a person has hypothyroidism. Symptoms of an underactive thyroid can include fatigue and weight gain. This condition should be diagnosed and stabilized with a prescription thyroid hormone prior to starting The OWL Diet.

Less commonly, people may develop an overactive gland with excessive release of thyroid hormones. Patients who have this condition, called "hyperthyroidism," often report unexpected weight loss. This condition also must be diagnosed, treated, and stabilized before starting a weight-loss program.

Treatments for all thyroid conditions must be continued during The OWL Diet. Losing weight will not affect the dose of the medications that you are taking.

Arthritis

There are many forms of *arthritis,* but the most common type is called osteoarthritis (OA), which affects weight-bearing joints such as the knees and hips.

Risk factors for OA include previous joint injury (trauma), age, family history, and obesity. Weight-bearing joints bear the burden of supporting and carrying the extra pounds associated with obesity. Over years, that burden leads to wear and tear of those joints. Cartilage thins out and bony spurs form around the joints. Eventually, the "shock-absorbing" cartilage disappears and joints become "bone-on-bone." At this point the OA is severe and associated pain and reduced mobility leads to the need for joint replacement surgery.

With successful weight loss on The OWL Diet, many people report a reduction in joint pain. Certainly the control of obesity at any stage in life will have positive effects on how your joints will feel and how well they function for you.

Sleep Apnea

Obesity may contribute to snoring and *sleep apnea*. Fatty tissue may accumulate in the neck. This may in turn lead to partial obstruction of the airway when sleeping. This is especially a problem when we sleep on our backs. The snoring that results may be disruptive to our relationships. Snoring may also be a sign of a more serious underlying problem called "sleep apnea." During sleep apnea, there are pauses in breathing with drops in the levels of oxygen that is carried to the heart and brain. Sleep apnea is diagnosed by a sleep study and may be treated by devices that assist in keeping the airway open during sleep.

With weight loss, snoring and sleep apnea frequently improve. If you have been prescribed a device to use for sleep apnea, such as CPAP (continuous positive airway pressure), then you should keep using it while you are losing weight. After successful weight loss, consult with your doctor to see if a repeat sleep study is needed to determine if the device is still needed. Do not stop treating sleep apnea without receiving medical advice first.

Infertility

There are many causes of *infertility*, but as a general statement it can be said that obesity can affect hormone levels in women, and this can affect the regularity of the menstrual cycle and reduce fertility.

Polycystic ovary syndrome (PCOS) is part of a broader condition recognized as metabolic syndrome (formerly syndrome X) that occurs more commonly in overweight individuals. One feature of this condition is reduced fertility. Loss of unwanted fat can, in certain cases, improve fertility in women with PCOS.

However, while you are on The OWL Diet, we want you to use contraception because a low-calorie diet is not advised for pregnant women. HCG (human chorionic gonadotropin), one of the prescribed therapies that may be used on The OWL Diet, is also the hormone whose levels we are looking for in pregnancy tests. Even though the dose of HCG used for weight loss is very small, it may trigger a false positive pregnancy test (a positive pregnancy test in the absence of actual pregnancy). As stated in chapter 4, if you believe that you may have become pregnant while on The OWL Diet then you must stop the diet immediately, discontinue use of HCG for forty-eight hours, and then take another pregnancy test.

If you are using low-dose HCG to assist in your weight-loss program, be aware that the low dose of HCG will not increase your fertility nor will it interfere with your use of hormonal birth control such as the birth control pill.

Cancer

Obesity has been established as a risk factor for certain cancers, including breast and endometrial (uterine) cancer. Losing weight will reduce the risk for some individuals.

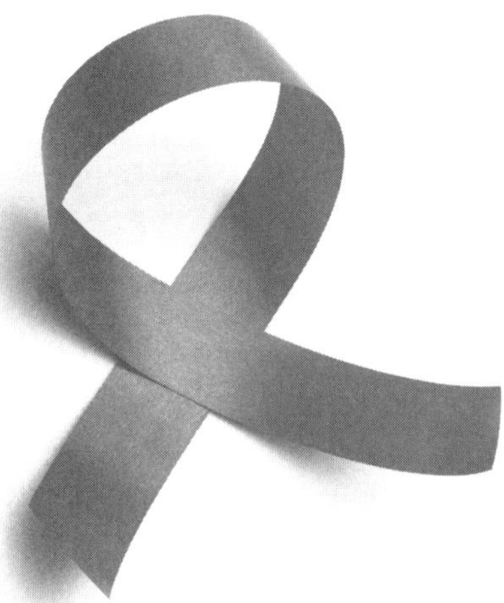

Cancer survivors can participate in The OWL Diet plan.

When a history of cancer already exists, then you need to discuss the possibility of your following The OWL Diet with your oncologist (cancer expert). You may be advised not to use HCG therapy, even in low doses. You should be able to safely follow The OWL Diet with the use of other or no OWL prescription medications.

I suggest that men who have had prostate or testicular cancer and women who have had breast cancer avoid the use of HCG.

Neurologic Disorders

The nervous system comprises the brain, spinal cord, and all nerves in the body. Many different medical conditions may affect the nervous system. The effects of some diseases may also impact the level of an individual's physical activity. Some conditions that can affect physical activity are:

- Multiple sclerosis
- Stroke
- Nerve damage (neuropathy) from spinal cord injury

Individuals with these conditions are at increased risk of becoming overweight or obese due to their lack of physical activity. It is very important for these people to work to maintain as much mobility as possible. Ultimately, these individuals must learn to eat healthfully to avoid developing weight problems. On The OWL Diet, they will not lose weight as quickly due to their reduced levels of physical activity.

Gall Bladder Problems

Inflammation of the gallbladder is called *cholecystitis*. It typically leads to the surgical removal of the gallbladder. Obesity is one of the risk factors for cholecystitis.

Ironically, in the era of bariatric surgery (weight-loss surgery), there is also a clear indication that rapid weight loss can trigger a gallbladder problem.

With The OWL Diet, the rate of weight loss is typically slower than that seen with successful bariatric surgery. As a result, my experience has been that development of a gallbladder problem while on my low-calorie diet is uncommon.

I inform my patients that a gallbladder problem may occur at any time in their life, and may therefore occur while they are on any diet or not dieting at all.

Irritable Bowel Syndrome

Irritable bowel syndrome (IBS) is a very common condition affecting men and women. Symptoms of IBS can vary from constipation to diarrhea, or a combination of both. Patients often complain of excess bloating, cramping, and increased flatus (gas).

When people follow The OWL Diet, they are eliminating most processed foods and all dairy products. The result is that the majority of people with IBS report less bloating, less abdominal discomfort, and less flatus. Some patients have reported that their IBS has gone away as long as they continue a healthful eating pattern.

I lost twenty-nine pounds! I reached my goal weight and have maintained my weight loss. To me, this experience wasn't a diet—it was a program that helped me develop good habits and stay accountable.
Jay, 35

I have seen some patients with IBS who suffered from severe constipation before starting The OWL Diet. These patients require special consideration. On The OWL Diet your bowel movements will typically become less frequent. Patients who are normally very regular before dieting may become constipated on a reduced-calorie diet. If a person suffers from constipation before starting The OWL Diet, they require medical advice that may lead to the use of calorie free fiber supplements, stool softeners, and laxatives as needed.

GERD

GERD is an abbreviation for *gastro-esophageal reflux disease.* In this condition, stomach acid migrates into the esophagus. The human esophagus is not designed to handle the acidity of stomach acid. The presence of stomach acid that refluxes into the esophagus can cause symptoms of chest pain, burning, or discomfort. Over time, continued acid exposure may result in changes to the lining of the esophagus that may cause narrowing (strictures) or cellular changes (Barrett's) that may in turn lead to esophageal cancer.

Although GERD is caused by several factors, there is no question that abdominal obesity creates a mechanical pressure on the stomach that increases the risk or severity of GERD. As a result, weight loss is often associated with an improvement in this condition, with fewer symptoms and possibly less need for medication to treat GERD.

A group of medications called proton pump inhibitors (including Nexium, Prilosec, and Prevacid) reduce stomach acid production and are often prescribed for GERD. When used daily, these medications have been demonstrated to adversely affect the absorption of vitamin B-12, increase the risk of pneumonia and certain forms of diarrhea. In these patients, use of supplemental vitamin B-12 by injection once to twice per week is very important while they are on The OWL Diet.

11

Maintenance: Keeping the Weight Off

You may be reading this chapter before you even start The OWL Diet. You may need some reassurance that you will keep the weight off after you have worked so hard to lose it. Perhaps you have had success with other diet plans, only to gain all the weight back. What was the point of dieting? You will be glad to know that I agree with you. A diet is only a success if it teaches you how to keep the weight off. Permanent weight loss is the goal of all OWL Diet participants.

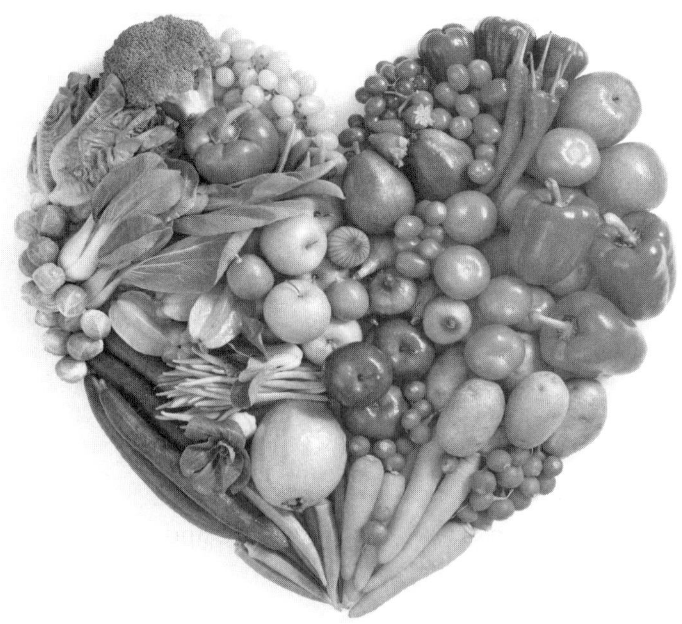

I believe that "yo-yo" dieting is more prevalent when you lose weight using protein powders, shakes, and prepackaged meals. Sure, these programs may work to help you lose the weight, but because it is unrealistic that you will keep buying their packaged foods indefinitely, invariably the weight all goes back on when you finish the program. Why is that? I believe that programs that sell you their food do not teach about healthful nutrition. Eating better, what I call food behavior change, is the cornerstone of keeping the weight off.

My maintenance plan is both simple and complex. The simple part is this: The OWL Diet will teach you to eat healthful food, in healthful portions throughout the day, and in maintenance you will need to continue to make healthful food choices. Most people then give me a skeptical look, suggesting that it is not a maintenance plan! People lose their skepticism after they see how well they do on the diet by eating real food. After two or three months of OWL dieting, most people realize they should continue to eat healthfully for the rest of their lives!

The complex part of my maintenance plan is that it truly is not easy to eat healthfully all the time. It is all too easy to relapse into old eating patterns and gain back the weight. The good news is that it's your choice. If you *decide* to keep the weight off, you can have total ownership of that decision. You can lose weight and keep it off.

Now let's move on to the point where you have successfully completed The OWL Diet and have reached your goal weight!

You Have Reached Your Goal Weight!

You worked hard to stay on The OWL Diet, but you stuck with it and reached your goal weight. You should feel a strong sense of accomplishment and empowerment from this success. Congratulations! You have once and for all taken control over your weight. You need to know that you now also have all the tools needed to maintain the weight loss. OWL dieting has taught you to enjoy healthful foods. You have learned that you can get by just fine with smaller portions. Now you need to continue this healthful way of eating for the rest of your life. I will not say that maintenance eating is easy—it is not. There will be times when you fall way off track, and then need to get back to the basics of eating The OWL Diet way.

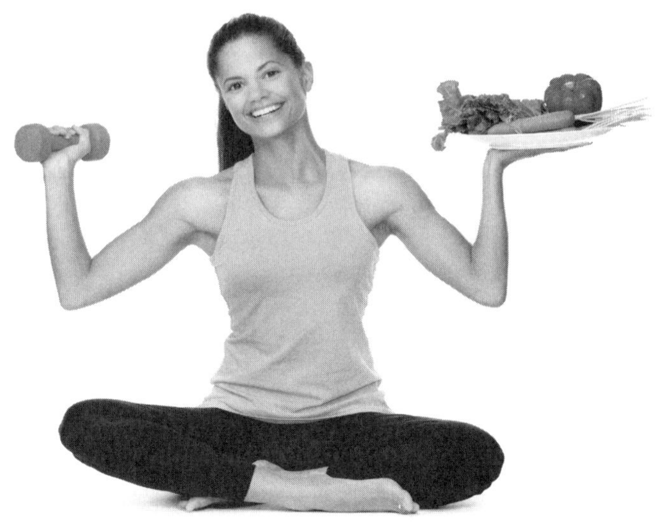

Maintain the weight loss by eating smaller amounts of lean healthful food, and with regular exercise.

Don't be surprised if you find yourself taking note of how other people are eating and notice that many are eating like you used to do! They may be eating fat, rich, oily food; portions that are too large; and too quickly. You will feel at times that no one else around you is eating healthfully the way that you are.

The reality is that most people in your life are a long way from making healthful food choices. Our society has a long way to go to solve the obesity problem. The good news is that you personally can choose to have total control over your weight.

Maintenance eating does not mean dieting for the rest of your life. In fact, if you continue to consume less than 1,000 calories per day, you will keep losing weight to the point that your BMI is too low, and your health is again at risk. You will likely be surprised at how much food you can now eat and not gain weight. But be careful testing out that theory!

I want you to become very protective of the pounds that you have shed. Don't allow yourself to go back to old eating habits. Don't regain the weight that you have worked so hard to lose! Be firm and stubborn in your resolve. The key is to eat healthful most of the time so that you can occasionally have a small amount of treats or foods that were avoided on the diet.

The 85/15 Plan: Eating Healthfully Six Days per Week

The OWL Diet has taught you to enjoy eating fresh fruits and vegetables and lean meats. Now you know to limit your intake of oils, carbs, and dairy products. You have also learned portion control. The OWL way of eating is a very healthful way for you to approach food.

Once you've reached your goal weight, The OWL Diet's maintenance plan allows you some flexibility to enjoy limited food treats that are not on the diet plan's approved list. I call this flexible maintenance program the 85/15 Plan. The 85/15 Plan is pretty simple. It is based on eating healthfully 85 percent of the time so that you can enjoy limited extra food and calories the other 15 percent of the time, with the goal of not gaining weight. I call the food consumed during the 15 percent of the time your food "treats." Another way of putting it is, 85 percent of the time you need to eat like a wise OWL and 15 percent of the time you can enjoy a few treats!

Treats, Not Cheats

If you followed the 85/15 model during the active weight-loss portion of The OWL Diet, you would be "cheating." Chances are, if you were like me, you tried this once or twice, just to see if you could get away with it! Believe me—you can't!

Of course, if you overdo it on calories during the 15 percent part of the plan, you will gain weight. There are limits to what you can eat. If you overdo it with food (and/or alcohol), you will be "cheating on your treats"! Overall, I believe you will be pleasantly surprised how many "treats" you can have 15 percent of the time and still maintain an appropriate weight.

Choose Days for Dieting and Days for Treats

In the 85/15 Plan, the 85 percent represents about six days of the week. During those six days you will follow the wisdom of OWL food selection and portion control. During the other one day per week, what I call the 15 percent treat time, you can enjoy a wider range and variety of foods. For the lovers of sweets and chocolates, this is the time worth waiting for every week!

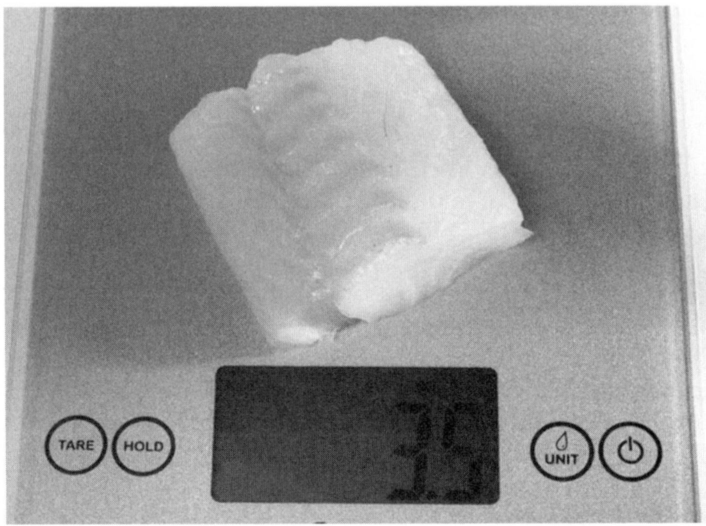

Continue to weigh your portions of protein. Seven ounces per day remains a healthful amount of meat or seafood in maintenance.

Or, the 85/15 Plan also gives you flexibility to choose when you can enjoy your extra food treats. Rather than one day per week, the 15 percent treat time can also be seen as three meals per week. With this interpretation, you can choose the three meals per week when you allow yourself to indulge in extra food and calories. By staggering the three meals out over the course of the week you may feel less deprived. You can also align these three meals with your travel, social, or business calendar.

OWL Maintenance Tips

During maintenance, you should still be eating three meals and three snacks per day, just as you did during active OWL dieting. Some foods should be avoided altogether. I like to say we retire them. They include deep-fried foods, French fries, potato-style chips, peanut butter, regular butter, and whipping cream. You may be able to think of a few others that you personally need to add to this list. But other than avoiding these taboos foods, maintenance of your weight loss is relatively easy and straightforward.

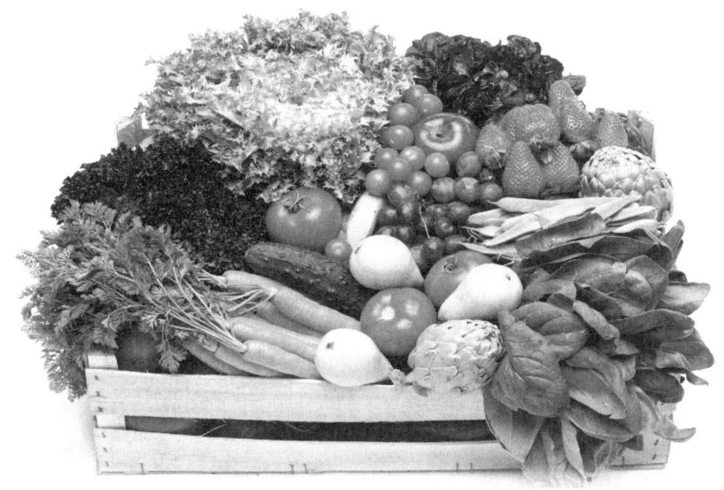

Continue to enjoy a wide variety of fresh vegetables every day.

Watch Portion Sizes

Keep your portions of meat small, and keep your meat lean. In the past, many of us consumed far more meat than we needed. Most days you will find that you do not need to consume more than seven ounces of any form of meat.

You may now enjoy small portions of pasta, rice, and potatoes. Smaller means about one-third of what you might have eaten in the past. I would not eat more than three servings of any of these starchy foods over an entire week.

Eat Lots of Fruits and Vegetables

Continue to eat lots of fresh fruits and vegetables. You may now also have pineapple and bananas, but not every day. When sweet corn is in season, enjoy one ear of corn, and then skip corn for a few days. You may now have dried fruits, remembering that the calories are concentrated and a small handful is more than enough.

Choose Healthful Nuts

The OWL Diet did not allow nuts, due to their high calorie count. You may now bring nuts back into your diet, but keep the portions small. Learn which are healthful nuts and which are unhealthful. I suggest that you choose almonds, pecans, and walnuts. Avoid peanuts in any form and honey-roasted nuts. Limit consumption of macadamia and cashew nuts, which are oily and therefore higher in calories.

Enjoy Limited Breads and Grains

On The OWL Diet, you had a small portion of bread or grain products daily. You can continue with bread and grains, but be very careful to not increase the portions too fast. Bread products are all high in calories, even the more healthful whole wheat and whole grain products. Brown rice may be more healthful than white rice, but it is still very high in calories.

Choose Egg Whites

Continue to limit your consumption of egg yolks, as they are very high in calories and cholesterol. Enjoy egg whites as much as you like.

Select Low-Fat Cheese and Dairy Products

You may also start eating any form of cheese. On The OWL Diet I did not allow cheese due to its high calorie count. Learn to slice your cheese into smaller pieces and eat them slowly. Cheese melted onto vegetables and meats is delicious, but not a good habit to start. Also avoid adding cheese slices to sandwiches. Check out the low-fat wedges of cheese, often packaged in silver foil; they make for great snacks and are low in calories. Also look for the small cheese rounds covered in red wax. These rounds are often only about fifty calories and make for a great snack.

Continue to eat yogurt, but choose the low-calorie, fat-free choices. If you tried almond milk on the diet, hopefully you liked the taste. Almond milk comes from a healthful nut and is high in calcium. Try to use low-calorie almond milk in place of cow's milk.

Keep Drinking Water and Limit Caloric Drinks

Continue to drink lots of water. Avoid high-calorie beverages such as regular soda pop and fruit juices. If you used to use cream in your coffee or tea, I suggest you avoid restarting

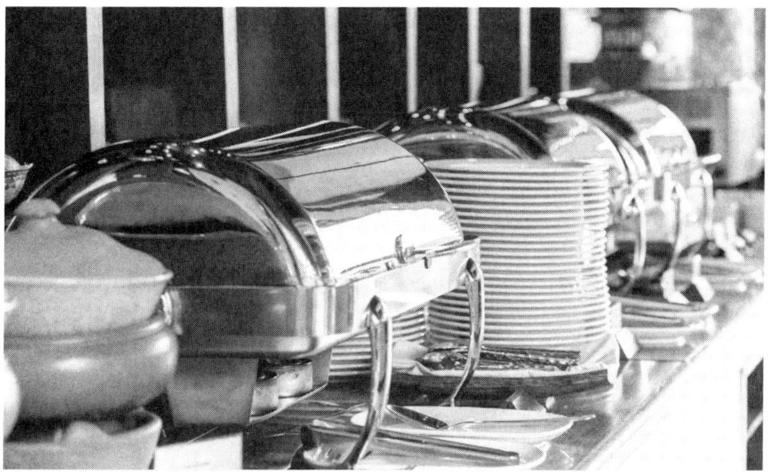

When dining in restaurants, the buffet is a "danger zone." Use what you have learned on the OWL Diet to make healthful choices.

its use. If you must use a creamer, choose a fat-free style and use as little as possible. Continue to limit your use of alcohol. All forms of alcohol are high in calories.

Beware of "Danger Zones"

By "danger zones," I mean foods that I believe can be very addictive. They include fast-food hamburgers and pizzas. If you love desserts, allow yourself the occasional indulgence, but try to keep the portions under control. I suggest that desserts and sweet treats need to be special indulgences, not daily events. Avoid bringing desserts and candy home. Resist eating unhealthful food that coworkers bring to the workplace.

Exercise Routine and Weight Watching

Exercise is important to helping you maintain a healthful weight. At a minimum, walk at least three days per week for thirty-minute intervals. If you want to be more physically active, then this is the time to start.

Weigh Yourself Daily

Weigh yourself every day. Your weight can fluctuate—there will be celebrations and special events. As a guideline, never allow yourself to gain more than three pounds over your goal weight. If you do gain more, focus on eating lower-calorie, lean foods in smaller portions, just as you did on the diet program. After one or two weeks of eating lean and healthful foods, you will see the pounds come off.

If You Gain Back Ten Pounds or More

As I have stated, permanent weight loss is a lifelong challenge and commitment. It is not easy, and there will be times in your life when you relapse into unhealthful eating patterns. There will be life-event stressors such as a divorce, changes in employment, financial strain, illness, loss of a loved one. The list goes on.

If your weight gets out of control and you gain ten or more pounds, then I suggest that you sign up for another month of the medically supervised OWL Diet. There is no shame in gaining the weight back. You will, of course, feel a sense of disappointment, but you must let that go and stop beating yourself up.

I have had many successful dieters come back for another month or two of OWL dieting for this reason. We are not here to judge you. We know you are as human as the rest of us. The important thing is to recognize that you need to refocus and benefit from the structure of The OWL Diet.

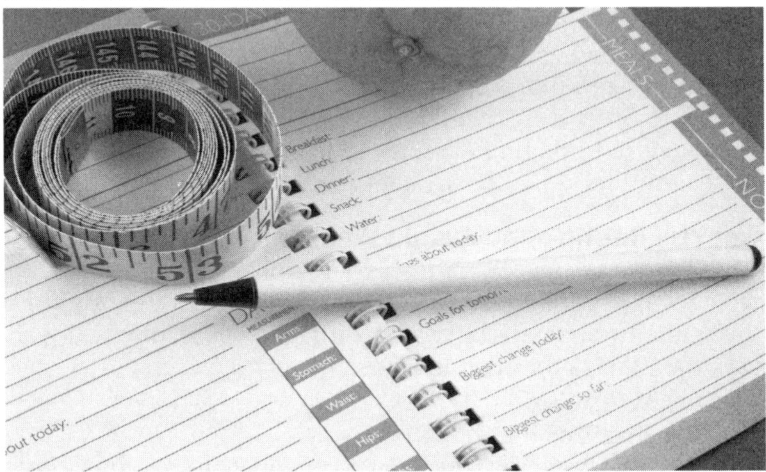

Weigh yourself daily and if you gain back ten or more pounds, come back and do another month of The OWL Diet.

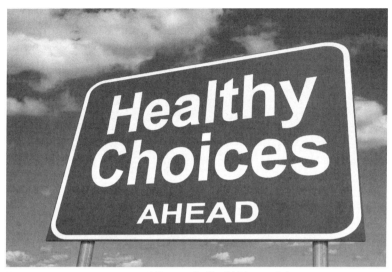

Maintenance eating is continuing to follow a path of healthful eating behaviors.

Maintenance Calorie Counting

There is not a magic calorie allowance per day that works for all people. The count will vary based on our gender, age, activity level, and metabolic rate. Furthermore, who wants to count calories every day for the rest of their life?

The better way to determine how much food you can eat is by weighing yourself every day. You will find out what foods work for you. If you gain three pounds, then you need to make some adjustments to the portions and food choices.

Helpful Eating Tips

- Eat your fruits whole and avoid drinking fruit juices. Eating the fruit of one California navel orange will provide about 65 calories. Compare that to just one cup of fresh or frozen orange juice that measures in at around 110 calories!
- Buy your vegetables fresh or frozen. Avoid canned vegetables that have lost much of their nutritional value and contain too much salt.
- Start your own garden and enjoy the satisfaction of growing and eating your own food. Community gar-

dens are a great choice for urban dwellers with limited green space. Have a balcony? Start a small container garden. You'll be surprised how much food you can grow in a small area!

- Support your local farmers and farmers' markets.
- Keep reading labels—look for "calories per serving" and "serving size" or "servings per container." By following this practice you will place many items back on the shelf!
- If you do not recognize the names of the top five ingredients of a packaged food, it's probably not good for you.
- Don't grocery shop when you are tired or stressed. You are more likely to make impulsive poor food choices.
- Shop the perimeter of the grocery store. This is where the real food tends to be placed: fruits, vegetables, meats, and dairy. Don't feel compelled to push your grocery cart up and down every aisle.
- Plan your meals for the week. The OWL Diet has taught you to organize and always have healthful food choices on hand.

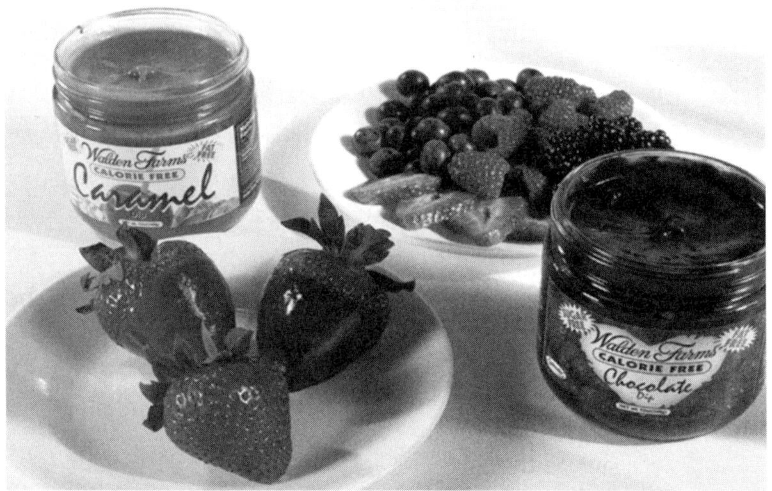

Keep using Walden Farms products that are calorie free, such as their chocolate and caramel dips.

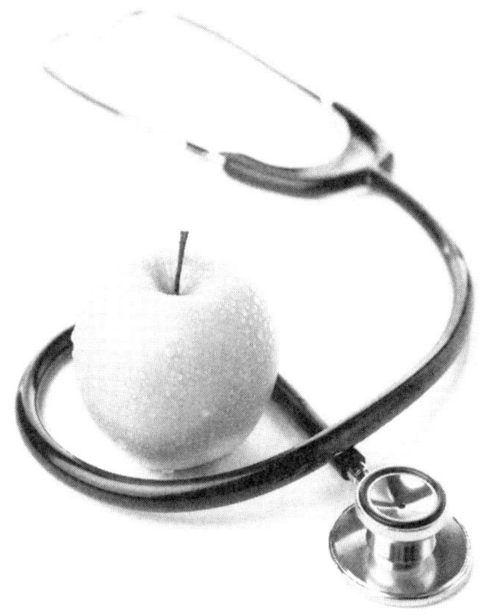

Your doctor is a part of your weight-loss team. Discuss any problems you're having, so he or she can help you succeed.

- Prepare meals in advance and always take food to work for lunch and snacks.
- If you choose to eat dairy products, as most of us do, go back to enjoying them in low-fat or fat-free forms, such as: skim milk, almond milk, fat-free yogurt, low-fat cheeses such as mozzarella, fresh goat, feta, grated Parmesan, and 1 percent cottage cheese.
- In America we tend to eat as though we are in a huge hurry. Slow down. Taste the food you eat. Savor the flavors. And stop eating before you feel completely full.
- When dining in a restaurant, consider an appetizer as your complete meal, or order an entrée and have the server place half of it in a take-home container before it even arrives at your table.
- Treats are just that—treats. They are not meant to be a part of your daily eating habit. Enjoy a dessert by following the 85/15 rule, and know there are limits.

- If you want ice cream, buy it in a small single serving from the grocery store. Pails are meant for sand castles, not for take-home ice cream.
- Try frozen yogurt or sorbets instead of fat-laden ice cream.
- If you want a cookie, buy a cookie, not a bag of them.
- Want a piece of pie? That's fine, but buy it by the slice and not the whole pie.
- Don't eat supper at the cinema. You should be going for the movie, not the popcorn.
- No more supersizing of anything!
- Avoid anything that looks like some form of chip—made from potatoes, corn, or other grains. The oil content is simply too high. By reading the calorie content on a bag of potato chips I'm sure you will agree.
- Choose olive oil for cooking, when oil is called for. Remember that 1 tablespoon of olive oil is approximately 120 calories! A small bottle should last a very long time.
- Continue to enjoy seasonings in your diet. Fresh lime and lemon juice can be freely used. Make Bragg Liquid Aminos your ongoing choice for soy sauce. Explore some of the other low-calorie/fat-free dressings that are now available to flavor your salads.
- Consider eating from smaller plates at home. The size of our dinner plate has actually increased over the past few decades, making us think we need to fill it up.
- Leave serving bowls in the cupboard. Dish up your food directly to your plate in the correct serving size. When you are finished, do not go back for seconds. Learn to love leftovers!

I am proud of you for taking control over your weight. Well done! You did it the natural and healthful way—with real food. And you have learned how to eat better. You can now lead a healthier life. You look better in the mirror, better in pictures, and better in your new clothes! Your confidence and self-esteem are at all-time highs! Congratulations!

12

Frequently Asked Questions about The OWL Diet

Over the years, I have noted recurring questions that OWL Diet participants raise during their weekly visits for coaching and support. Here are some of those questions, with my answers.

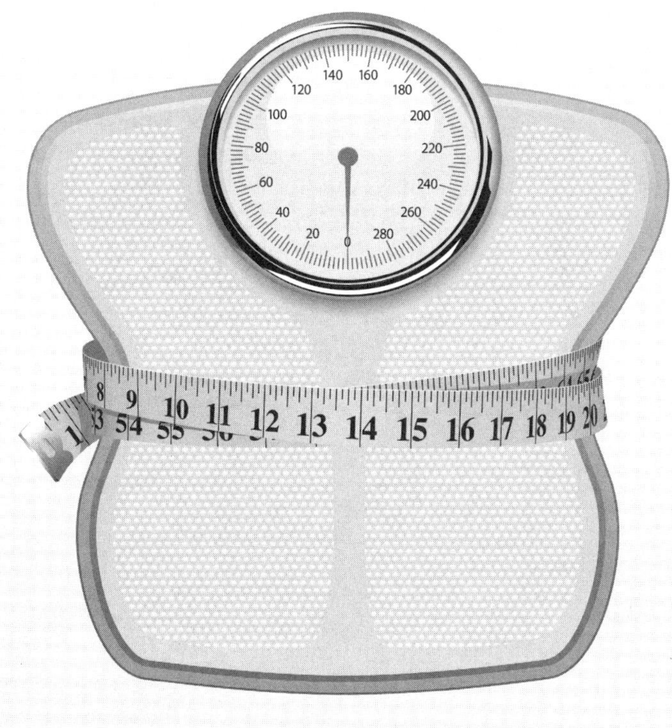

Why can't I go on a 500-calorie-per-day diet?

A diet limited to 500 calories per day is not safe. This is the calorie count of the original "HCG Diet," a diet that I think is far too restrictive in food choices and calories. Losing weight is not a race, it is a journey. The goal is to lose weight safely and keep it off for the rest of your life. If you starve yourself on only 500 calories per day, you will become weak and lose muscle mass as well as fat. I would predict that most people will gain all of the weight back after stopping such a restrictive diet.

Some days I get more calories than others. Is this OK?

Yes! I designed The OWL Diet to provide a great deal of flexibility of food choice. If you eat a wide range of approved foods, then you will be getting approximately 800 calories per day. You really do not have to count the calories of the food that I allow—I have already done it for you. Follow the portions, spread your food out over the course of the day, and you will have weight-loss success.

What can I eat if I don't like vegetables?

Vegetables are a necessary part of a healthful diet for everyone. There is no alternative to eating vegetables. I don't believe you can have a balanced diet without vegetables. There are many fresh vegetables readily available. You have to explore different ones and find some that you like. Compare the taste of them raw versus cooked. Try adding different seasonings to see if that will help. By cooking several vegetables together, the flavor also changes. Take that new flavor combination and mix it with your favorite meats such as lean beef or chicken.

It is interesting to note that most infants aged one to two love vegetables. At some point later on in childhood, people must get conditioned away from eating them. Chances are great that if you keep an open mind, your adult palate will guide you to vegetables that taste acceptable. You may even grow to like them a lot.

Will my bowels change while I am on The OWL Diet?

Almost everyone reports a change in their bowel pattern while on the diet. If prior to The OWL Diet you avoided fruits and vegetables, chances are that you will have some loose stools or diarrhea in the first two weeks of the diet. This will go away as your body adjusts to eating healthful foods.

If you have a history of irritable bowel syndrome, the most common report from OWL dieters is that this condition improves on the diet. I suspect this results from eating fresher, more healthful foods that are lower in oil, sugars, and additives.

Overall, the trend is that your bowel movements will be less frequent. If going every two to three days is comfortable for you, then there is no problem.

If, however, you are getting constipated, then action needs to be taken. Call or visit the health care provider working with you on the diet plan to discuss treatment options.

If you develop diarrhea that lasts for more than a week, then you should stop the diet and consult with your regular physician.

How do I manage persistent hunger?

Hunger is perhaps the greatest obstacle with any diet plan. The causes of hunger are very complex. We often eat not because we actually need to eat. As you follow The OWL Diet your hunger cravings should lessen. The stomach becomes smaller and you adjust to eating smaller meals. Always stay well hydrated. Eating calorie-free fiber with water can reduce hunger. Graze on your food throughout the day. Learn to chew your food thoroughly, and eat slower. The prescription medication phentermine works well to curb hunger, but not all people are able to take this medication.

Can a person prone to migraine headaches go on the diet?

Yes. One of the triggers for migraine headache can be hunger, or skipping a meal. The OWL Diet teaches you to eat several meals and snacks per day. This method of eating works well to avoid triggering a migraine due to hunger. Stay well hydrated, limit caffeine intake, and get enough sleep.

Can a person who has had breast cancer follow the plan?

Yes. If you have had breast cancer and you are obese you can reduce your risk of developing a recurrence of breast cancer by dieting to achieve an appropriate weight. There is often a connection between hormones and breast cancer, so it is important to talk this over with your doctor. My advice is to avoid using hormones if you have a history of breast cancer, despite the fact that there is no proven connection between use of and the development of breast cancer. Breast cancer survivors can take other medications such as phentermine and topiramate to help them succeed on the diet plan.

What can I eat if I don't like fruit?

The health benefits of fruit are great, and they should be used on the diet plan and for the rest of your life. Challenge yourself to explore fruit again. Try raw or cooked. Season your fruit with artificial sweeteners, lemon or lime. Try adding cinnamon. If you like yogurt, you can substitute an eighty-calorie cup of yogurt for one serving of fruit.

Can I take my own vitamins and supplements?

The OWL Diet Pack contains vitamins and supplements that have been carefully selected to work well on The OWL Diet plan. We include the cost of these supplements with your monthly fee to participate. It is our expectation that you will use them. The OWL Pack contains premium products that are produced in the United States under strict supervision. These supplements are free of lactose and additives. Do not take other multivitamins or B-complex vitamins with The OWL Pack. If your regular doctor wants you on additional doses of calcium or vitamin D, then these may be added to the OWL Pack, but only after medical consultation. You may use additional sources of fiber that are calorie-free.

Why can't I run while on The OWL Diet?

At an average of 800 calories per day The OWL Diet will provide you with enough energy to engage in normal day-to-day activities. We also allow mild to moderate physical activity, but that does not include running. It is not safe to run or exert yourself that hard while on a reduced-calorie diet. You may develop light-headedness, and you might even faint, causing bodily injury. Also, the hunger that is created from running or working out too hard is ravenous hunger that will lead to eating extra calories and failing the diet.

I am a woman who has gone through menopause. Vaginal spotting occurred while I was dieting. What should I do?

Use of even low-dose HCG during The OWL Diet has been rarely associated with vaginal spotting. If this occurs to you, and you have been in menopause for at least one year, then I suggest that you see your primary care doctor to report the problem. He or she may advise you to have an endometrial ultrasound or endometrial biopsy. Bleeding after menopause can be a sign of endometrial cancer. This form of cancer is not caused by The OWL Diet. In fact, losing weight will reduce your risk of endometrial cancer.

Will I lose hair from the top of my head on this diet?

Although losing hair is a common complaint with dieting in general, I can report that it is not a frequent complaint on The OWL Diet plan. I believe the reason for this is that I allow for an adequate intake of calories selected from a wide variety of healthful foods, and I provide a high quality OWL Diet Pack full of vitamins and supplements that nourish scalp hair growth.

What if I feel light-headed or dizzy?

Complaints of light-headedness or dizziness are usually due to low blood sugar, dehydration, or low blood pressure. On The OWL Diet you are encouraged to drink plenty of water, eat throughout the day, and monitor your blood pressure on a regular basis. As long as you follow these simple rules you should not have this problem. If you are on blood pressure medication, with weight loss a reduction in doses or even elimination of your BP medicine is commonly necessary. This decision should be made only by your health care provider.

Can I stay on my other medications?

Your health care provider will need a complete list of all of the medications that you are taking. He or she will make recommendations on whether you need to adjust or change any medications at the start of the diet, and periodically during your weight loss.

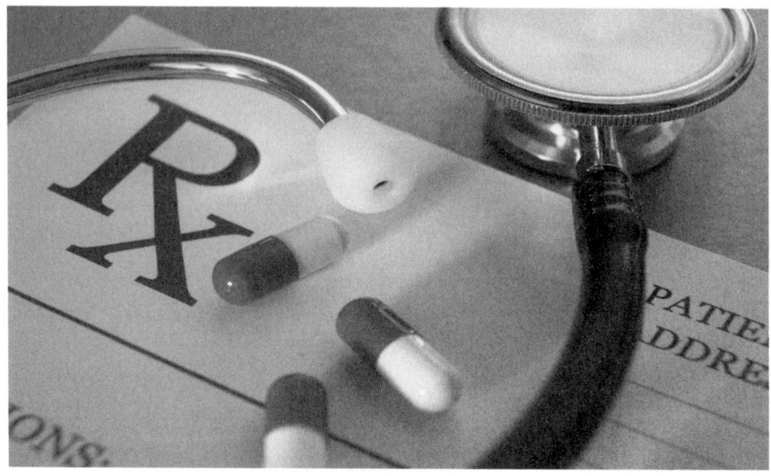

Tell us all medications that you are taking; some of them may need to be adjusted as you lose weight.

Can I stop my CPAP after I lose some weight?

Stay on CPAP (a device used for sleep apnea) while you are on The OWL Diet. It is true that weight loss can reduce the need for use of CPAP. However, it is important to continue nightly use of CPAP during your weight loss. Once you achieve your goal weight, your primary doctor will likely want to repeat your sleep study to assess whether you will continue to need CPAP or not.

Am I allowed to eat rice or pasta on the diet?

Rice and pasta are too high in calories and are not allowed on the diet. After you lose weight, you may resume periodic use of small amounts of rice and pasta.

Can I stop my cholesterol medication after I lose some weight?

Stay on your cholesterol medication while you are losing weight. After you reach your goal weight, then visit with your doctor who prescribes this medication to discuss your options. High cholesterol is often hereditary and you may need to stay on medication for the rest of your life.

What if I have a medical problem and cannot exercise?

People who are unable to walk or exercise can still participate in The OWL Diet. Try to be as active as you safely can. Your rate of weight loss may be slower than if you were able to exercise, but you will lose weight. With weight loss, perhaps your ability to be active will improve.

My job is very physically active. Will I need to eat more food?

You may need to eat more food if your job involves a great deal of physical activity. Take extra approved food to work with you. I suggest that you try one or two extra servings of fruit if necessary. If you need to take in extra calories, always take food that is OWL Diet approved.

My family is not supportive of my efforts to lose weight. What can I do?

It is disappointing when your family is not supportive of your desire to achieve an appropriate weight. You may ask yourself why that is. Are they overweight? Are they always negative? The good news is that you can do this without their support. You cannot change your family or their attitudes. But you can decide to take total control over your weight! Follow the diet and you will succeed.

What about other foods that are not mentioned on the diet?

Over several years I have added more food variety to The OWL Diet plan. I did this to make the diet easier for people to have success with, prevent food boredom, and smooth the transition from dieting to maintenance eating. If a food is not mentioned on The OWL Diet list of approved foods, then do not try it. Attempts at tweaking the diet are almost always met with failure to lose weight.

As the food industry starts to respond to the need for low-calorie, low-fat food options we are starting to see more selection. If you find a new food item that you think should work, please discuss it first with your health care provider who is working with you on The OWL Diet before trying it on your own.

Am I allowed to eat nuts on the diet?

Nuts are not allowed on the diet. They are too high in calories. You will see in chapter 11 that nuts are allowed as part of maintenance eating, but with a few basic rules to follow.

What can I safely take to help me get to sleep?

There are several options. One of the most common "sleep aids" is over-the-counter diphenhydramine, which is better known by the brand name Benadryl. As a sedating antihistamine, diphenhydramine is often taken at night. It helps some people get to sleep quicker but may cause some drowsiness and dry mouth the next morning.

Another option is to take the hormone melatonin, also available over the counter in an oral pill form. Your brain naturally produces melatonin and levels often rise prior to going to sleep. By taking additional melatonin one hour before bedtime, it may help you to get to sleep more easily. Some people who take melatonin report a side effect of undesirable dreaming.

If you are already taking a prescribed hypnotic then discuss continuing the use of this medication with your health care provider.

Will taking The OWL Diet plan's prescribed medications interfere with my birth control pill?

None of the five prescribed treatments currently used with The OWL Diet will have any effect on the birth control pill. The most common cause of failure of "the pill" is missing a dose.

What if I think that I might be pregnant while on the diet?

OWL dieters should take adequate precautions to prevent pregnancy. If you believe that you may be pregnant it is important to stop The OWL Diet and resume normal eating. If you are taking any of the prescribed medications used with The OWL Diet, they should also be discontinued at this time. If you have been using HCG, you must wait forty-eight hours from the last dose before performing a pregnancy test. If you are pregnant, contact your physician immediately to initiate prenatal care.

I am having leg cramps. What can I do?

There are several possible causes of leg cramps. If you are not consuming enough fluids, cramping may occur. Another cause is related to the acidosis that occurs when dieting. During acidosis the body shifts potassium. Although your total body potassium may not have changed, your muscles may perceive a potassium deficit and cramping may occur. Less commonly, muscle cramps are from varicose vein disease, or a side effect of medication. Cholesterol medications that are part of the "statin" family can also cause this side effect. Discuss your leg cramping with your health care provider to determine the cause and solution.

I am scheduled to have surgery. Should I stay on the diet?

I suggest that you discontinue dieting and the use of diet-related prescriptions at least two weeks prior to surgery. Resume a diet of healthful food with a normal amount of calories. After you have recovered from surgery, and have the permission of the surgeon, you may resume The OWL Diet.

Can I take breaks from the diet, and if so, for how long?

After two months of continuous dieting, many participants take a break for anywhere from a week to a month. During this time you will discontinue use of prescription-diet medications, such as phentermine. Read chapter 11, "Maintenance: Keeping the Weight Off," for helpful suggestions on making healthful food choices during your break so that you do not gain weight back.

Breaks may also be taken for one day only, such as during a birthday, celebration, graduation, anniversary, or holiday. Longer breaks are allowable when you are on vacation. Taking breaks on the diet will not interfere with your progress once you restart the diet plan. Think of your eating patterns during breaks as practicing how to eat in maintenance.

Business travel can also be a good time to take a break. If you attend meetings where food is provided, take great care to avoid foods that will result in a weight gain. Conferences are notorious for serving unhealthful foods at breakfast and during breaks.

In Closing

The OWL Diet changed my life, and my wife's life as well. I am so pleased that this realistic program of eating healthfully has helped so many other people, and I hope that it will continue to have a positive impact on many other people's lives.

With this updated version of The OWL Diet I have focused on the importance of medical supervision while on a reduced-calorie diet. I have expanded my list of prescription treatments (medications and hormones) that are now available and can help you achieve your personal weight-loss goal. I made a conscious effort to reduce the emphasis on the use of HCG, which is no longer a cornerstone of The OWL Diet plan.

I have also provided a longer list of vitamins and supplements that we now use with The OWL Diet program, including a grain-free fiber, garcinia cambogia, and linoleic acid.

I have also added to the variety of food options that are allowed while dieting. Yogurt and almond milk are now part of The OWL Diet's food options. The OWL Diet today results in an average intake of 800 calories per day, creating a further distance from overly strict and unsafe 500-calories-per-day diet plans used in the past.

I now understand more about the complex interplay between our emotional health and our ability to make changes in the way that we eat. I have incorporated some behavioral modification techniques to help participants ask themselves some of the tough questions about motivation to change their weight, and how to get past emotional roadblocks.

Stay connected with further developments on The OWL Diet at **www.OWLDiet.com.**

Appendix

Instructions for Injections of HCG

The "gold standard" for administering HCG is to do so by injection. It's the way I personally administered the HCG to lose my weight. In the United States, HCG is always obtained by prescription that is then dispensed by a pharmacy. As a prescription medication in the United States, HCG hormone is labeled to be given by injection into muscle (intramuscularly). The following instructions are based on injection of HCG into the thigh muscle.

HCG for injection is sold as a sterile powder in glass vials. The powder will need to be converted into a liquid for injection. This step is called "reconstitution." Either your pharmacy will reconstitute HCG for you, or you will be directed how to do this at home. HCG is reconstituted using bacteriostatic water. A specific measured amount of bacteriostatic water is drawn up by syringe and injected into the vial of sterile HCG powder. The powder should dissolve into a clear liquid without difficulty. Once the HCG is reconstituted it must kept in a refrigerator where it is stable and usable for the next sixty days.

On The OWL Diet, the standard dose of HCG by injection is 125 IU (international units) administered intramuscularly, once every morning, seven days per week for four continuous weeks (one cycle). After a four-week cycle is completed, if additional weight loss is needed, then a second four-week cycle may begin immediately.

For home injection you will need the following supplies that you may obtain from your doctor or pharmacist:

- single-use alcohol prep pads
- cotton balls
- bandages
- biohazard container, also called a "sharps container," for safe storage of used needles and syringes
- single-use, sterile syringes and needles

Most people find it quite easy to learn how to self-inject medications. The average person also reports the discomfort of injection to be minimal. I suggest you use the following technique for daily HCG injections:

- Wash and dry your skin at the injection site to be sure it is clean and free of lotion or cream.
- Wash your hands thoroughly with soap and warm water.
- Sit on a chair or on the side of the bed with your feet flat on the floor.
- Use a single alcohol prep pad to first clean the rubber stopper on your bottle of HCG, then use the same alcohol prep pad to clean your skin on the front (top) part of your thigh over the large muscle called the quadriceps.
- Use a cotton ball to dry the alcohol.
- Remove a new syringe and needle from its packaging. With a twisting motion, make sure the needle is securely attached to the syringe.
- Pull the cap off the needle and pull back on the syringe plunger, drawing air into the chamber of the syringe to equal the amount of HCG solution that will be injected.
- Insert the full length of the needle into the HCG vial and inject the air. Invert the vial and pull back on the plunger, filling the syringe with the correct daily dose.
- Hold the loaded syringe in your hand like a writing pen.
- With your hand no more than three inches (eight centimeters) from your thigh, point the needle at a ninety-degree angle (perpendicular) to the skin. Use a wrist action, and with one smooth motion confidently

inject the needle into the muscle. Make sure the entire length of the needle is inserted into the skin. The discomfort should be minimal.

- If there is excessive pain on insertion, the needle may be too close to a small nerve. If so, pull out the syringe and reinsert into a new location.
- Holding the syringe with both hands, carefully pull back slightly on the plunger. If blood appears in the clear HCG fluid, you're in a vein, and the needle should be removed without injection and placed into an alternate location.
- Once you are satisfied you're not in a vein, inject the HCG slowly, taking about five seconds to empty the syringe.
- Leave the needle in the thigh for another five to ten seconds to allow the fluid to absorb.
- Remove the needle from your thigh. Do not recap the needle onto the syringe. Discard the needle and syringe, attached to each other, into a suitable biohazard container.
- Apply light pressure at the injection site with the cotton ball and apply a bandage if desired.

The risks of injection include discomfort, bruising, or development of a skin infection at the injection site. See your health care provider right away if any redness or inflammation occurs at the injection site; this may be a sign of infection.

Instructions for Using Transdermal HCG Cream

Not everyone is comfortable with or able to learn self-injection. The good news for them is that the success of hormone absorption across the skin has been well documented. This form of absorption is called "transdermal." Creams and gels used for administration of other hormones such as testosterone, estrogen, and progesterone. I have used HCG transdermal cream with very good results in my OWL Diet patients.

This product is available by prescription from compounding pharmacies. HCG is blended into a rapid absorbing cream by the pharmacist. It is typically dispensed in a "compounding cream syringe" that has a cap on the end. HCG cream may be safely stored at room temperature, or it may be refrigerated. HCG cream is not stable when exposed to bright light or high temperatures. Many people store this product in the bathroom drawer at normal room temperature and away from light.

Ask your pharmacy regarding the proper technique that they recommend when transferring cream from the syringe to the inner forearm.

HCG transdermal cream is applied in a dose of 125 IU once per day in the morning. The simplest choice for men and women alike is to apply a measured dose of the cream to the inner forearm.

I suggest you use the following technique:

- Remove watches and bracelets from both forearms.
- Wash and dry your hands and forearms using soap and water to ensure they are clean and free of any other oils or creams.
- Apply the measured dose of HCG cream to one inner forearm. Then rub both forearms together until the cream is absorbed (about one minute). Avoid putting other cream, lotion, or sunscreen on this area for one hour.
- Women may use the breast or inner thigh instead of the forearm. Men should avoid hairy areas, so the inner forearm is often their best choice. Hair on the inner forearm may be shaved off prior to application of the HCG transdermal cream.

Index

About the Author

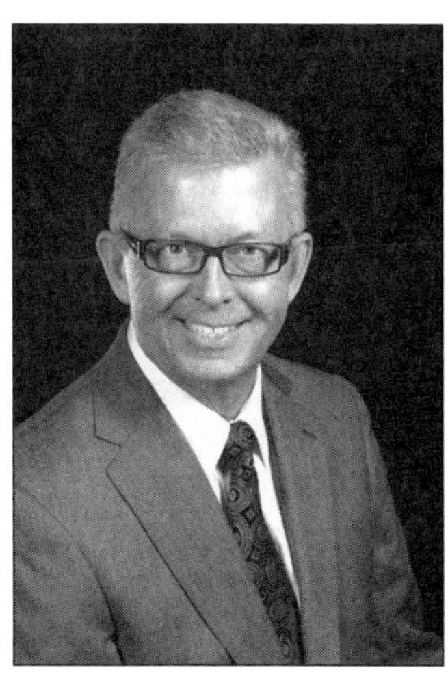

Carter O. Abbott, M.D., is the medical director of the Omaha Med Spa, in Omaha, Nebraska, which he opened in 2006. During his own quest for a weight-loss plan, Dr. Abbott developed the Omaha Weight Loss Diet, known as "The OWL Diet," and he has helped hundreds of patients succeed in losing weight. Dr. Abbott also specializes in nonsurgical aesthetics as part of the Med Spa services.

Dr. Abbott received his medical degree from the Schulich School of Medicine at Western University in London, Ontario, Canada, and completed postgraduate training in family medicine at St. Joseph's Health Centre, London, Ontario, Canada. A primary care physician in both Canada and the United States for more than thirty years, Dr. Abbott's work has taken him to both urban and rural settings. He has practiced in clinics, hospitals, nursing homes, palliative care facilities, urgent care clinics, and emergency rooms. Dr. Abbott's diverse experience has equipped him with a unique understanding of the obesity problem that faces many of us today.

To reach Dr. Abbott and to stay up to date on The OWL Diet, please visit: **www.OWLDiet.com.**